Advanced Nursing Practice and Nurse-led Clinics in Oncology

Over the past ten years, there has been a dramatic increase in new nursing roles and nurse-led clinics within oncology. This unique handbook is a comprehensive companion for nurses studying and practising at an advanced level in this emerging field.

This text outlines and discusses roles, responsibilities and skills related to advanced practice in oncology nursing – including leadership, communication skills and prescribing – linking throughout to the implications for clinical practice. It then provides a step-by-step guide to setting up and developing nurse-led clinics, looking in more detail at clinics focusing on surgery, chemotherapy, radiotherapy, clinical trials and follow-ups, and providing an in-depth case example of a clinic set up for adjuvant Herceptin use.

Practical, relevant and underpinned by current legislation, *Advanced Nursing Practice and Nurse-led Clinics in Oncology* is an invaluable resource for oncology nurses.

Carole Farrell is a Nurse and AHP Research Fellow at the School of Oncology, the Christie NHS Trust, Manchester, UK. She is Honorary Lecturer at the University of Manchester, UK.

Advanced Nursing Practice and Nurse-led Clinics in Oncology

Edited by Carole Farrell

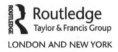

Routledge
Taylor & Francis Group

LONDON AND NEW YORK

First published 2016
by Routledge
2 Park Square, Milton Park, Abingdon, Oxon OX14 4RN

and by Routledge
711 Third Avenue, New York, NY 10017

Routledge is an imprint of the Taylor & Francis Group, an informa business

British Library Cataloguing-in-Publication Data

A catalogue record for this book is available from the British Library

Library of Congress Cataloging-in-Publication Data
Advanced nursing practice and nurse-led clinics in oncology / edited by
   Carole Farrell.
      p. ; cm.
   Includes bibliographical references and index.
   I. Farrell, Carole, editor.
   [DNLM: 1. Neoplasms—nursing.   2. Advanced Practice Nursing—
methods.   3. Oncology Nursing—methods. WY 156]
   RC266
   616.99'40231—dc23
   2015007728

ISBN: 978-0-415-74649-6 (hbk)
ISBN: 978-0-415-74650-2 (pbk)
ISBN: 978-1-315-79750-2 (ebk)

Typeset in Times
by Apex CoVantage, LLC
Printed in Great Britain by Ashford Colour Press Ltd,
Gosport, Hants

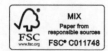

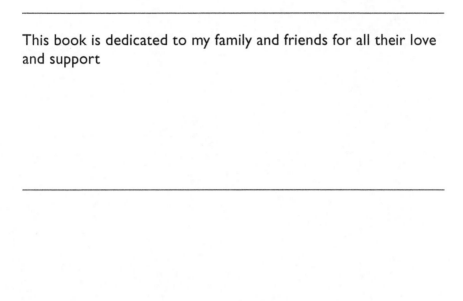

This book is dedicated to my family and friends for all their love and support

Contents

Tables and figures

TABLES

FIGURES

BOX

Preface

My current role is a nurse and AHP research fellow in the School of Oncology at the Christie NHS Trust, which involves initiating and running academic nursing research studies. My main research interests are around the impact of cancer and anti-cancer treatments from patients' and carers' perspectives, and also nurses' clinical roles and nurse-led clinics, therefore working with clinical nurses and allied health professionals (AHPs) is very important to me when developing research proposals and translating findings into clinical practice. My PhD focused on exploring oncology specialist nurses' roles and an ethnographic study of nurse-led chemotherapy clinics. My main aims from nursing research are to improve patient and carers' experiences, and enhance the delivery of clinical services. Within this I am very keen to help nurses and AHPs develop their research skills and undertake non-medical research projects. I am also an honorary lecturer at The University of Manchester, and Consultant Editor of *Cancer Nursing Practice*.

I have worked in oncology for almost thirty years, working on surgical, radiotherapy and chemotherapy wards, including haematology and bone marrow transplantation units. My roles have also included chemotherapy sister, research sister (clinical trials) and five years as a clinical nurse specialist (CNS) in breast cancer. Whilst working as a CNS I also had two part-time secondments at The University of Manchester, as a nurse researcher and a lecturer practitioner, which expanded my academic skills.

In 2003 when I became a nurse clinician (advanced nurse practitioner) my main aims were to improve continuity of care for patients and develop nurse-led clinics. Working across clinical and medical oncology was challenging at times but provided scope for developing nurse-led models of care and continuity for patients. As a nurse clinician my role had similar clinical responsibilities as the specialist registrars; I would see similar patients and be expected to manage them in the same way as a doctor, including new patients. My medical responsibilities included history-taking, clinical examination, prescribing, ordering investigations and interpreting the results. I was able to admit and discharge patients, reduce doses of chemotherapy or stop treatment due to excess toxicities or suspected progressive disease, although this was usually in collaboration with the medical consultant.

In addition I would discuss treatment options, including potential clinical trials, with patients and their family, undertake symptom management, management of their cancer and elements of supportive, social and psychological care. I saw patients at all stages of breast cancer and oncology treatment: neo-adjuvant, adjuvant, metastatic/palliative, which also included identifying patients within the last 12 months of life and discussing advanced care planning and preferred place of care with patients in the terminal stage of their illness. I worked closely with the breast care nurse specialists, referring patients to them when patients required a greater level of psychological, social or financial support that I could provide in clinic, however this required careful negotiation to avoid stepping on their toes. I also worked closely with the specialist palliative care nurse during end of life care or complex pain management.

Throughout my role as a nurse clinician I was more interested in continuity of care and improving patients' experiences. This fuelled my drive to develop nurse-led clinics, which I began in 2004. Further details of this, with examples from my clinical practice, are documented within this book to illustrate how nurse-led clinics can be set up, including different types of nurse-led clinics and models. I have also included some tips and suggestions based on my own experiences, which readers may find helpful.

Contributors

Dr Carole Farrell PhD, MPhil, MSc, MA, RGN Nurse and AHP Research Fellow, School of Oncology, the Christie NHS Trust, Manchester. Honorary Lecturer, the University of Manchester

Alison Franklin MEd, BA (Hons), Dip Couns, Dr Claire Green PhD, BSc (Hons), Nicola Schofield MPhil, BSc (Hons) Senior Trainers, Maguire Communication Skills Training Unit, School of Oncology, the Christie NHS Trust, Manchester.

Dr Elaine Lennan PhD, MSc, RGN Consultant Chemotherapy Nurse and Health Education Wessex Fellow, University Hospital Southampton.

Helen Roe MSc, BSc (Hons), RGN Consultant Cancer Nurse, North Cumbria University Hospitals

Introduction

This book aims to focus on advanced nursing practice in oncology, including nurses' roles and nurse-led clinics.

There have been significant changes to nurses' roles and responsibilities in the last decade leading to role expansion, the development of new roles and advanced levels of nursing practice. However, this has often created confusion due to the plethora of nursing titles and myriad of different specialist roles within oncology nursing. This will be addressed by providing a timeline of oncology nursing developments alongside changes to professional regulations and discussing the impact of relevant cancer policies. Explanations and discussions will be clear, relevant and underpinned by current legislation to outline current implications for clinical practice.

Subsequent chapters will outline current frameworks for oncology nursing, discussing nurses' roles, responsibilities and associated competencies, and illustrating changes to professional boundaries. The implications surrounding the expansion of nurses' roles will be highlighted, discussing potential tensions that may arise within or between professionals, and strategies for success will be outlined.

The expansion of nurses' roles has required nurses to undertake additional training and achieve clinical competencies. Generally non-medical prescribing and clinical examination skills are essential requirements within advanced nursing practice, alongside communication skills and additional role-specific skills. This book will outline how such skills have changed the face of advanced nursing practice, and enabled nurses to extend clinical services to benefit patients.

Over the past ten years there has been a dramatic increase in nurse-led clinics within oncology. However, there are wide variations in the nature of nurse-led clinics and the scope of nurses' clinical practice. Many nurse-led clinics have arisen ad hoc in response to local demands, and nurses often lack guidance in setting up and running nurse-led clinics. This book aims to provide a step-by-step approach towards setting up and developing nurse-led clinics, discussing current professional and policy implications for nurse-led clinics, legal issues and nurse prescribing.

This book will provide a useful resource for oncology nurses which is up to date, relevant and evidence-based. Written by nurses who have a great deal of

Table 0.1 Operational definitions

Nursing title	Operational definition
Specialist nurse (clinical nurse specialist)	Nurses who specialise within a specific condition or treatment pathway
Advanced nursing practice	A level of practice beyond initial registration
Advanced nurse practitioner	Nurses with advanced level skills and knowledge, working in a specialist or a generalist area within primary, secondary or tertiary care.
Oncology clinic	An outpatient clinic for patients with cancer
Chemotherapy clinic	An outpatient clinic for patients undergoing chemotherapy
Nurse-led clinic	An outpatient clinic that is run or managed by registered nurses
Nurse-led chemotherapy clinic	An outpatient clinic for patients undergoing chemotherapy that is run or managed by registered nurses

experience within advanced nursing practice and nurse-led clinics, this book will cover operational issues with examples from clinical practice in different settings.

Given the lack of clarity regarding specialist and advanced nursing roles, and also different interpretations of nurse-led clinics, the following operational definitions will be used (see Table 0.1). Whilst some operational definitions are clearly defined in the literature, the remainder are outlined by the author where definitions are elusive.

Chapter 1

Nursing developments and policy influences

Carole Farrell

This chapter provides a timeline for professional developments in nursing, including a brief discussion on nursing models, alongside discussions of influential government policies. Emphasis will be placed on developments in oncology nursing and cancer policies. This will provide a historical summary of developments, outlining the major factors to impact on nursing roles. Implications for service provision and the impact of government targets and quality measures will be discussed to show how this has influenced nurses' roles and responsibilities.

However, in order to understand nurses' roles it seems crucial to consider current operational definitions for nursing, specialist and advanced nursing practice, and nurse-led clinics. This seems particularly important given the confusion created by the plethora of nurses' titles and clinical roles.

Defining nursing

What is a nurse? It seems such a simple question, but when you actually focus on it there are differences in meaning and imprecise definitions. In some ways, when you look at the history of nursing and how it has evolved, the lack of precision seems understandable, particularly since the main component of nursing is 'caring', which is rather vague and lacking in scientific rigour. This makes it difficult to quantify and measure what nurses do within their roles; as a result, determining outcomes from nursing becomes complex and often requires qualitative analysis. To ensure clarity it seems crucial to peel back the layers of nursing and discuss basic definitions and meanings within nursing.

The International Council of Nurses (ICN) states that the title of 'nurse' should be protected by law and applied to and used only by those legally authorised to represent themselves as nurses and to practice nursing (ICN, 2012, 2013). However, in the UK there is no legal definition of nursing, although a legislative definition for 'registered nursing care' is in place to distinguish between other types of care, such as social care (RCN, 2003). In contrast, most countries have a legal definition of the title 'nurse' and some have a legal definition of 'nursing', although the definitions and scope of practice vary from country to country. It seems difficult to comprehend the lack of consensus in defining nursing at its most basic level;

however from this basis it seems unsurprising that we are struggling nationally to define advanced nursing practice.

However the following broad definition of nursing is provided by the ICN (2014):

> Nursing encompasses autonomous and collaborative care of individuals of all ages, families, groups and communities, sick or well and in all settings. Nursing includes the promotion of health, prevention of illness, and the care of ill, disabled and dying people. Advocacy, promotion of a safe environment, research, participation in shaping health policy and in patient and health systems management, and education are also key nursing roles.

Nursing care usually refers to the tasks and activities of the nurse, and often reflects everything a nurse does for a patient (DalPezzo, 2009). Although there are many attributes of nursing care, there appear to be three main categories:

- The tasks or procedures
- The nature of nursing care (for example skilled, compassionate, holistic)
- The functions of nursing care (for example, listening, assessing, monitoring) (DalPezzo, 2009)

These categories reflect different aspects of nurses' roles and are important factors to consider when exploring what nurses do within clinical practice.

Nursing models

Nursing models were developed in order to define nursing and to provide a framework to guide practice and education (Murphy et al., 2010). A nursing model is a collection of interrelated concepts or components that can be taken apart and understood, and all nursing models involve assessing patients' needs and implementing appropriate care. However the components of nursing are complex and difficult to define; therefore several models were created, each offering a different way of thinking to guide nursing practice (Murphy et al., 2010). (See Table 1.1.) However it is crucial to include goals that can be measured or evaluated to determine future improvements. The majority of nursing models utilise care plans that can be evaluated daily to record each patient's progress; however there are a range of different theories within nursing models, and most are no longer used within current nursing practice.

The original nursing role incorporated a biomedical model of care, which was prescribed by a physician and focused on physical aspects of care and the treatment of disease. Before the development of nursing models nurses used the medical model, which focuses on diagnosis and treatment of specific illnesses or conditions (Murphy et al., 2010). Alternatively nurses relied on their intuition and experience. However, the biomedical model does not take into account individual characteristics such as ethnicity, culture, and religion. This contrasts with a social

Table 1.1 Nursing theorists and nursing models

Nurse theorist	Name of model	Main concepts
Florence Nightingale (1859)	Environmental theory	• Unsanitary conditions pose a health hazard. • Nursing can provide fresh air, warmth, cleanliness, good diet, quiet to facilitate reparative process. • External influences can prevent or contribute to disease or death.
Hildegard Peplau (1952)	Interpersonal relations model	• The person is a developing organism, tries to reduce anxiety caused by needs, lives in a stable equilibrium. • Based on psychodynamic nursing. • Uses an understanding of one's own behaviour to help others identify their difficulties. • Nursing is a significant, therapeutic, interpersonal process that functions cooperatively with others to make health possible, and involves problem-solving.
Ida Orlando (1961)	Deliberative nursing process	• The deliberative nursing process is set in motion by the patient's behaviour. • All behaviour may represent a cry for help. Patient's behaviour can be verbal or nonverbal. • The nurse reacts to patient's behaviour and forms basis for determining nurse's acts. • Nurses' actions should be deliberative, rather than automatic. • Deliberative actions explore the meaning and relevance of an action.
Dorothy Johnson (1980)	Behavioural systems model	• The person is a behavioural system comprised of subsystems constantly trying to maintain a steady state. • Constancy is maintained through biological, psychological, and sociological factors. • A steady state is maintained through adjusting and adapting to internal and external forces. • Nursing is an external regulatory force that is indicated only when there is instability.
Dorothea Orem (1991)	Self-care model	• Self-care comprises those activities performed independently by an individual to promote and maintain person well-being. • Self-care deficit occurs when the person cannot carry out self-care. • The nurse then meets the self-care needs by acting or doing for; guiding, teaching, supporting, or providing the environment to promote patient's ability. • Wholly compensatory nursing system – patient dependent. • Partially compensatory – patient can meet some needs but needs nursing assistance. • Supportive educative – patient can meet self-care requisites, but needs assistance with decision making or knowledge.

(Continued)

Table 1.1 (Continued)

Nurse theorist	Name of model	Main concepts
Betty Neuman (1982)	Health care systems model	• The person is a complete system, with interrelated parts. • Maintains balance and harmony between internal and external environment by adjusting to stress and defending against tension-producing stimuli. • Nursing interventions strengthen flexible lines of defence, strengthen resistance to stressors, and maintain adaptation.
Sister Calista Roy (1980)	Adaptation model	• The person is an open adaptive system with input (stimuli), who adapts by processes or control mechanisms (throughput). • The output can be either adaptive responses or ineffective responses.
Roper, Logan, Tierney (1980)	Activities of daily living model	• The patient is assessed on their ability to perform the 12 activities of daily living. • The goals of the care plan are agreed between patient and nurse, then evaluated. • 5 dimensions: physiological, psychological, socio-cultural, politico-economical, environmental.
Maslow (1970)	Hierarchy of needs model	• A 5-stage model based on a person's needs, placed in a hierarchy. • Stages go from basic (physiological) needs to safety needs, social needs, and esteem needs, with self-actualisation being the highest level. • Later expanded to an 8-stage model to include cognitive and aesthetic needs, with transcendence needs (helping others to achieve) at the top.
Patricia Benner (1984)	From novice to expert model	• Describes 5 levels of nursing experience and developed exemplars and paradigm cases to illustrate each level. • Levels reflect movement from reliance on past abstract principles to the use of past concrete experience as paradigms, and change in perception of situation as a complete whole in which certain parts are relevant.

model of health care which emphasises potential changes within society or life-style factors that may improve health.

The emergence of nursing models aimed to develop a broader focus based on human needs and developing therapeutic relationships with patients (McCrae, 2012). However, nursing theorists have struggled to provide precise definitions for nursing and achieve consensus regarding theoretical nursing models.

All models have four elements: the person, their environment, their health, and nursing (Fawcett, 1995); and nursing models have three key components:

- A set of beliefs and values
- A statement of the intended goal
- The knowledge and skills required (Pearson et al., 1996)

Although all models have a different emphasis, they are influenced by the following continuums:

- Optimum health   Ill health
- Independence   Dependence
- Adaptation   Maladaptation
- Self-care   Reliance on others

Nursing models/theories emphasise a more holistic approach to disease, although the term 'holistic' is often misused and open to interpretation (Farrell, 2014). However, models are not facts; rather they emerge and evolve, informing thinking and imply different nursing processes.

In the 1970s, the concept of the nursing process was introduced in the UK, which was a four-stage model incorporating assessment, planning, implementation, and evaluation (MacFarlane and Castledine, 1982). However, the introduction of patient pathways and standardised multidisciplinary approaches became the gold standard from the 1990s to emphasise quality in health-care provision (Currie and Harvey, 2000).

Nursing models have been criticised for their frequent use of jargon and complex concepts, which led to problems in understanding (Hodgson, 1992; Kenny, 1993). In addition, some of the models developed in the USA appeared inappropriate for health systems in the UK (Murphy et al., 2010), or appeared to have narrow perspectives that failed to capture the meaning of nursing (Hardy, 1982). Despite seeking to articulate the nature of nursing as a discipline, the models seemed idealistic and increased the gap between theory and practice (Hardy, 1982). Models also lacked research underpinning the relationship between the concepts and impact on patient care (Fraser, 1996; Dickoff and James, 1968), and the application of nursing theories (Draper, 1990).

The emergence of nursing models aimed to develop a broader focus based on human needs and developing therapeutic relationships with patients (McCrae, 2012). However, nursing theorists have struggled to provide precise definitions for nursing and achieve consensus regarding theoretical nursing models.

More recently Wimpenny (2002) described three types of models, which seems a more simplistic approach:

- Theoretical: Developed by one person using inductive and deductive processes; presented as a picture of the reality of nursing; are aids to problem-solving within a paradigm, and to challenge nurses' ideas and concepts.
- Surrogate: A functional version of the theoretical model. Represents a framework for nurses to collect data and communicate.
- Mental: A personal schema of an individual nurse, built from knowledge and experience.

However, this still suggests a conceptual or theoretical approach to explaining nursing and lacks practical application; therefore in reality it is unlikely that this would be used by clinical nurses.

The development of nursing and dependence on doctors over the years has led to nurses adopting a subordinate role to doctors, often being regarded as a doctor's handmaiden (McCrae, 2012). Aggleton and Chalmers (2000) suggest that this will continue unless nurses value the unique contribution that they make to health care. This is an important point in relation to understanding nurses' roles and changes to nurses' clinical practice, since there are recent examples where medical consultants control what nurses can and cannot do in nurse-led clinics (Farrell, 2014).

Some of the theoretical models also failed to resonate with clinical practice, since they appeared to focus more on documentation rather than clinical nursing care. In addition, the availability of different theoretical models created conflict in determining the most appropriate model for nurses within clinical practice, and this lack of consensus may have led to their demise. This contrasted with medicine, where a single medical model focused on diagnosis, treatment, and curing physical disease. Although previous nursing models failed to bridge the gap between nursing theory and practice in the 1970s and 1980s (McCrae, 2012), there is now a move to rejuvenate nursing theory (Pridmore et al., 2010). More recently the introduction of care pathways in the UK changed the direction towards multidisciplinary approaches to care, which emphasised quality in service provision (Currie and Harvey, 2000).

However rising health-care demands and shortages of medical and nursing staff have led to new models of clinical care delivery and new operational models of nursing care (Dubois et al., 2012). A major factor driving changes to nurses' roles in the UK was the European Working Time Directive, which was introduced in 1993 and considerably reduced the working hours of junior doctors (Goddard et al., 2010; Pickersgill, 2001).

Policy context and service demands

The nursing profession, along with other health professionals and health services, is heavily influenced by government policies, legislation, and professional guidelines. In oncology this has shaped our clinical services, introducing priorities within the health service to improve patient care and ensure services are cost-effective. This continues to bring challenges in meeting government targets, such as waiting times; however it has also created opportunities for nurses to develop their roles and change the way they work to meet clinical demands. Whilst this chapter cannot cover every policy or guideline, it will provide a broad policy context for oncology nurses and discuss the main issues.

Cancer remains the biggest cause of premature death in adults under 75 years old, despite reductions in cancer mortality (DH, 2007). To address this, the government introduced a National Cancer Plan (DH, 2000a) that aimed to improve the efficiency and effectiveness of cancer services, and a Cancer Reform Strategy (DH, 2007), which emphasised the importance of high quality services reflecting patients' needs. However, the increasing incidence of cancer, and an ageing population, has huge implications for the National Health Service (NHS) to meet government targets and ensure high quality cancer services that are tailored to meet patients' needs (Cox et al., 2006).

Government policies have been instrumental in changing the directions of the NHS and influencing service delivery through mandatory directives. However, whilst the focus on targets, such as two-week waiting times for patients with suspected cancer, resulted in earlier diagnosis for some patients (Cox et al., 2006), there were some negative consequences. Firstly, this immediately placed the rising demands on existing clinical services and stretched clinical resources, since many hospitals were already working at full capacity. Secondly, clinicians were under pressure from hospital managers to meet targets, which focused on patient numbers and throughput rather than individuals. Thirdly, the drive to meet targets moved attention away from patients' experiences and the quality of service provision (DH, 2007).

The turnaround came in 2008 with the government's realisation that patients should be put first, by greater choice and emphasis on quality of care (DH, 2008), with subsequent recommendations to measure health outcomes rather than process targets (DH, 2010a). This also reflects the definition of quality set out by Lord Darzi in that high quality care comprises effectiveness, patient experience, and safety (DH, 2008), and this has been enshrined into the recent Health and Social Care Act 2012 (DH, 2012a). To achieve this aim the Darzi review (DH, 2008) set out to ensure that the NHS has a professional workforce that can meet demand, offer quality assurance for patients and their families, and meet demands set by health service commissioners.

The current NHS Outcomes Framework 2013/14 focuses on measuring health outcomes (DH, 2012b), aiming to act as a catalyst to drive quality throughout the NHS within five domains (DH, 2012b):

1. Preventing people from dying prematurely
2. Enhancing quality of life
3. Helping people recover from ill health

4. Ensuring that people have a positive experience of care
5. Treating and caring for people in a safe environment and protecting them from avoidable harm (DH, 2012b)

The five domains also resonate with the philosophy of cancer nursing.

Policy influences on oncology nursing practice

Several cancer policy documents have included key recommendations for clinical staff, leading to pivotal developments in cancer nurses' roles (DH, 1999a, 1999b, 2000a, 2007, 2008). *Making a Difference* outlined a need for nurses to work in different ways by extending nurses' skills and clinical roles (DH, 1999b). This was echoed in the National Cancer Plan (DH, 2000a), which proposed redesigning cancer services to make the best use of health professionals' skills. Emphasis was also placed on the need to introduce new service models for cancer (DH, 2007), and the potential benefits of nurse-led clinics and services (DH, 2008). However, whilst the policies open new directions for cancer services and provide resounding support for nurse-led clinics, they fail to provide any recommendations or strategies to develop and evaluate clinical and nurses' roles and nurse-led services. This is a crucial omission in ensuring the quality and effectiveness of nurses' roles and nurse-led clinics.

Alongside these government policies, professional policies were also introduced, which reviewed service provision and 'skill mix' within cancer nursing (DH, 2006; 2000b), aiming to clarify clinical leadership as well as individual roles and responsibilities (Bolton and Laycock, 2006). However, the Chief Nurse of England also emphasised the importance of nursing values, stating that 'patients want to feel safe, cared for, respected and involved', recognising the value of nurses who 'can combine technical skills with a deep understanding and ability to care', which highlights the value base, or essence, of nursing (DH, 2006 p4).

The Royal College of Nursing (RCN) (2007) proposed a need to redefine nurses' roles and careers, promoting unambiguous job titles with streamlined role definitions. In addition the RCN began developing professional nursing career pathways with four levels of practice, ensuring links with future demands for nursing care (RCN, 2007). However in reality the ad hoc development of new cancer nursing roles has created confusion and there is little evidence of evaluation. Unless new nursing roles are carefully evaluated, it seems difficult to appreciate their impact and effectiveness on patients and cancer service delivery, which may lead hospital managers to question their value.

There are certainly tensions between government policy, clinical demands, and nurses' roles where nurses seem to be pulled in different directions, which highlights their flexibility but also exacerbates their vulnerability. For example, the Cancer Reform Strategy (DH, 2007) recommends greater flexibility within the NHS and innovative ways of working to benefit patients, which opens an important pathway for nurse-led clinics and new models of clinical practice. However, despite this recognition, cost-cutting exercises have reduced some specialist nursing posts (Sullivan and Elliot, 2007; Kelly and Trevatt, 2006), which creates vulnerability amongst specialist nurses (Kelly and Trevatt, 2006). The survey by Farrell et al. (2011) also reported that nurses expressed uncertainties regarding their future professional roles within the NHS. Despite placing clinical nurse specialists at the forefront of modernising health care, playing a crucial role in improving the quality of cancer care, and being an essential part of the multidisciplinary team (MDT), Sullivan and Elliott (2007) warn of the danger that the role of the clinical nurse specialist (CNS) may be seen as a luxury. Considering the valuable work of clinical nurse specialists in oncology, this is worrying.

Ensuring 'value for money' and quality of care

One of the most fundamental aspects within the Cancer Reform Strategy is the need to ensure quality of care within service provision (DH, 2007). However there is also a strong emphasis on providing 'value for money' within cancer service delivery, and this may become the local driver for nurse-led services within NHS hospital trusts. Therefore it seems important that issues of quality are not lost within this process. In considering the satisfaction of patients, the Cancer Reform Strategy pledges to reduce pledges to invest more money in services that make a difference to patients (DH, 2007). Therefore, in terms of evaluating nurse-led services, it seems crucial to identify potential differences from patients' perspectives between nurse-led and medical management. This seems particularly important given that a further pledge from this policy document is to focus cancer spending on cost-effective interventions that make a difference to patients (DH, 2007). This is important given the current disparity between nurses' and doctors' pay, since the substitution of doctors by specialist nurses may be utilised as a cost-cutting exercise. However, the need to develop clinical nurse specialist roles and introduce advance nurse practitioners and independent prescribers should primarily be in order to improve patients' experiences; included in this is the need for 'successful' nurse-led follow-up (DH, 2007).

Summary

The rapid growth in nurse-led models of care and clinical cancer management certainly reflect service development opportunities within cancer policy documents (NAO, 2001). Indeed, reducing waiting times for patients has been one of the main drivers in the introduction of nurse practitioners and nurse-led clinics in order to meet local and national targets. However, it also seems important to focus on how cancer nurses have developed their practice; consider what training, support, and infrastructure are provided for role developments; and explore how service developments may have affected patients and service delivery. If nurse-led services are set up as a substitute for medical management, it seems crucial to evaluate their effectiveness and acceptability to patients.

Cancer policies have clearly set out a comprehensive strategy for improving cancer services in the UK. This aims to eradicate the 'post code lottery' and ensure patients have equality of access to high quality cancer services and increasing choice (DH, 2000a, 2007, 2008). However, government targets for new referrals and first treatment have placed a huge burden on service providers to see new patients and deliver cancer treatments within tight deadlines. Given the current financial pressures within the NHS, and the increasing costs of cancer treatments, this has tremendous implications for service delivery and clinical management.

The reduction in junior doctors' hours forced the NHS to look at redesigning the workforce to meet the clinical needs of patients and provide appropriate clinical management to address the reduction in medical staff (Ferguson and Kearney, 2000). At the same time, the nursing profession made plans to allow nurses to extend their roles and take on some of the tasks that were previously within the doctors' domain. Changes to nursing regulations have revolutionised the scope of professional nursing practice, increased nurses' autonomy, and led to a higher level of advanced nursing practice, with many nurses running clinics and services independent of medical staff.

The advent of nonmedical prescribing has made a fundamental improvement in increasing nurses' autonomy to provide a more comprehensive and holistic package of care for patients (Stenner and Courtenay, 2008a, 2008b; Courtenay et al., 2007). A significant number of nurses are now prescribing independently for patients, which has paved the way for more nurse-led clinics with the potential for greater continuity and increased choice for patients, as well as meeting government and hospital targets (Stenner and Courtenay, 2008b; Farrell and Lennan, 2013). Considering the disparities between medical and nursing salaries, this move also seems favourable to hospital trusts in their bid to provide cost-effective services.

However, despite the advances in nursing practice and improvements in nursing legislation to support it, there is a current lack of clarity regarding competencies for advanced practice and no clear role definition for advanced nurse practitioners. This is exacerbated given the plethora of nursing titles and lack of clear definition and regulation for the use of new titles, such as nurse practitioner and advanced nurse practitioner, which may cause confusion for patients, the public, and other health-care professionals. From this it seems important to explore more fully the concept of advanced nursing practice and new roles within it.

Similarly, although there has been a rapid growth in nurse-led clinics, there seems to be a gap in the legislation surrounding them, with a lack of clarity in definition, training, and competencies. Although some work has been undertaken on evaluating advanced nursing practice and nurse-led clinics, this seems limited, particularly within oncology. It seems that more work is needed to explore the concept of nurse-led clinics and consider the scope of nurse-led clinics within oncology. Although the driver for nurse-led clinics may be cost-effectiveness, it seems important to consider the impact on patients and existing services.

References

Aggleton P, Chalmers H. (2000). *Nursing models and nursing practice*, 2nd ed. Basingstoke, Macmillan.

Bolton E, Laycock W. (2006). Introducing skill mix to palliative care. *Cancer Nursing Practice*. 5(6): 20–24.

Cox K, Wilson E, Heath L, Collier J, Jones L, Johnson I. (2006). Preferences for follow up after treatment for lung cancer: assessing the nurse-led option. *Cancer Nursing*. 29(3):176–187.

Courtenay M, Carey N, Burke J. (2007). Independent, extended and supplementary nurse prescribing in the UK: A national questionnaire survey. *International Journal of Nursing Studiesa*. 44(7): 1093–1101.

Currie VL, Harvey G. (2000). The use of care pathways as tool to support the implementation of evidence-based practice. *Journal of Interprofessional Care*. 14(4): 311–323.

DalPezzo K. (2009). Nursing care: A concept analysis. *Nursing Forum*. 44(4): 256–264.

Department of Health. (2012a). *Health and social care act*. London, DH.

Department of Health. (2012b). *The NHS outcomes framework 2013/14*. London, DH.

Department of Health. (2010a). *Equity and excellence: Liberating the NHS*. London, DH.

Department of Health. (2008). *High quality care for all: NHS next stage review*. London, DH.

Department of Health. (2007). *The cancer reform strategy*. London, DH.

Department of Health. (2006). *Improving patients' access to medicines: A guide to implementing nurse and pharmacist independent prescribing within the NHS in England*. London, DH.

Department of Health. (2000a). *The NHS cancer plan*. London, DH.

Department of Health. (2000b). *The nursing contribution to cancer care*. London, DH.

Department of Health. (1999a). *Making a difference: Strengthening the nursing, midwifery and health visiting contribution to health and healthcare*. London, DH.

Department of Health. (1999b). Nurse midwife and health visitor consultants: Establishing posts and making appointments. *Health Service Circular* 218. Leeds, NHS Executive.

Dickoff J, James P. (1968). A theory of theories: A position paper. *Nursing Research*. 17(3): 197–203.

Draper P. (1990). The development of theory in British nursing: Current position and future prospects. *Journal of Advanced Nursing*. 15: 12–15.

Dubois CA, D'Amour D, Tchouaket E, Rivard M, Clarke S, Blais R. (2012). A taxonomy of nursing care organization models in hospitals. *BMC Health Service Research*. 12: 286–301.

Farrell C. (2014). *An exploration of oncology nurse specialists' roles in nurse-led chemotherapy clinics*. Unpublished PhD thesis, University of Manchester. Available at www.escholar.manchester.ac.uk/uk-ac-man-scw:224894 [accessed 16.02.2015].

Farrell C, Lennan E. (2013). Nurse-led chemotherapy clinics: Issues for the prescriber. *Nurse Prescribing*. 11(7): 561–566.

Farrell C, Molassiotis A, Beaver K, Heaven C. (2011). Exploring the scope of oncology specialist nurses' practice in the UK. *European Journal of Oncology Nursing*. 15(2): 160–166.

Fawcett J. (1995). *Analysis and evaluation of conceptual models in nursing*. Philadelphia, FA Davis Co.

Ferguson A, Kearney N. (2000). Towards a European framework for cancer nursing. In *Cancer nursing practice: A textbook for the specialist nurse* (N. Kearney, A. Richardson, and P. DiGiulio, eds.), pp. 179–196. Edinburgh, Churchill Livingstone.

Fraser M. (1996). *Conceptual nursing in practice*. London, Chapman Hall.

Goddard A, Hodgson H, Newbery N. (2010). Impact of EWTD on patient: Doctor rations and working practices for junior doctors in England and Wales. *Clinical Medicine*. 10(4): 1–6.

Hardy LK. (1982). Nursing models and research – a restricting view. *Journal of Advanced Nursing*. 7: 447–451.

Hodgson R. (1992). A nursing muse. *British Journal of Nursing*. 1(7): 330–333.

ICN. (2014). *Definition of nursing*. Available at http://www.icn.ch/who-we-are/icn-definition-of-nursing/ [accessed 16.02.2015].

ICN. (2013). *Scope of nursing practice*. Available at http://www.icn.ch/images/stories/documents/publications/position_statements/B07_Scope_Nsg_Practice.pdf [accessed 16.02.2015].

ICN. (2012). *Protection of the title nurse*. Available at http://www.icn.ch/images/stories/documents/publications/position_statements/B06_Protection_Title_Nurse.pdf [accessed 16.02.2015].

Kelly D, Trevatt P. (2006). NHS finances. *Cancer Nursing Practice*. 5(8), 14–18.

Kenny T. (1993). Nursing models fail in practice. *British Journal of Nursing*. 2: 133–136.

MacFarlane J, Castledine G. (1982). *A guide to the practice of nursing: Using the nursing process*. London, CV Moseby.

McCrae N. (2012). Whither nursing models? The value of nursing theory in the context of evidence-based practice and multidisciplinary health care. *Journal of Advanced Nursing*. 68(1): 222–229.

Murphy F, Williams J, Pridmore, JA. (2010). Nursing models and contemporary nursing 1: Their development, uses and limitations. *Nursing Times*. 106: 23.

National Audit Office. (2001). *Inpatient and outpatient waiting in the NHS: Report by the comptroller and auditor general*. London, DH.

Pearson A, Vaughan B, Fitzgerald M. (1996). *Nursing models for practice*. Oxford, Butterworth-Heinemann.

Pickersgill, T. (2001). The European working time directive for doctors in training. *British Medical Journal*. 323: 1266.

Pridmore JA, Murphy F, Williams A. (2010). Nursing models and contemporary nursing 2: Can they raise standards of care? *Nursing Times*. 106: 22–25.

Royal College of Nursing. (2007). Ensuring a fit for purpose future nursing workforce. London, RCN.

Royal College of Nursing. (2003). *Defining Nursing*. London, RCN.

Stenner K, Courtenay M. (2008a). The role of inter-professionals relationships and support for nurse prescribing in acute and chronic pain. *Journal of Advanced Nursing*. 63(3): 276–283.

Stenner K, Courtenay M. (2008b). Benefits of nurse prescribing for patients in pain: Nurses' views. *Journal of Advanced Nursing*. 63(1): 27–35.

Sullivan A, Elliot S. (2007). Assessing the value of a cancer clinical nurse specialist. *Cancer Nursing Practice*. 6(10): 25–28.

Wimpenny P. (2002). The meaning of models of nursing to practising nurses. *Journal of Advanced Nursing*. 40: 346–354.

Chapter 2

The changing face of oncology nursing

Carole Farrell

Leading on from the initial context of policy and professional regulations, this chapter will discuss the scope of nurses' roles and responsibilities, explaining the different ways that nurses' roles have expanded and extended, outlining the training requirements, and discussing the implications for clinical services and patient care. One of the key implications of nurses expanding their current roles is legislation; therefore it seems important for nurses to understand the potential impact on professional accountability when nurses increase their clinical/medical responsibilities.

Scope of practice

The scope of nursing practice is defined as 'the range of responsibilities which fall to individual nurses . . . related to their personal experience and skill' (UKCC 1992 cited in RCN 2003 p9). This is based on the premise that the limits of nursing practice should be determined by the knowledge and skills required for safe, competent performance, rather than a list of tasks or functions that nurses may or may not perform (RCN 2003). However, nursing is often defined by what nurses do, which is expressed in terms of their roles, functions, or tasks (RCN 2003). The difficulties of using this approach are highlighted by changes to nurses' roles over time, including changes to professional boundaries where nurses take on medical tasks and responsibilities. Similarly, some of the tasks traditionally undertaken by registered nurses are now completed by healthcare assistants or assistant practitioners.

Developments in nurses' roles have been ad hoc (Folland 2000), with variability across the UK, in Europe, and also worldwide (Bryant-Lukosius et al., 2004). Henderson (2006) explains that nurses' training and professional role varies within and between countries, although nurses may have the same title. Nevertheless, the lack of regulation in the UK regarding nurses' titles, role development, competencies, and responsibilities causes considerable confusion (Gardner et al., 2007).

The Royal College of Nursing (RCN) (2003) proposes that the ability of nursing to respond to people's needs depends on the way:

- nursing work is organised in healthcare delivery systems
- practice is regulated and the quality of care is assured

- practitioners are prepared
- nursing is defined

In addition each nurse is held accountable for their actions, which is outlined in the Code of Conduct (NMC 2008), and governed by the Nursing and Midwifery Council (NMC).

Expanding nurses' roles

It is clear that government policies and professional regulations have paved the way for developments in nurses' roles, enabling nurses to legitimately take on additional clinical responsibilities and practice within their professional guidelines. However, the major influence on how nurses' roles have expanded seems to be the increase in clinical demands and reduction in junior medical staff (Farrell 2014). Upskilling nurses to take on some of the traditionally medical tasks and responsibilities seems a convenient solution to plug some of the gaps in service provision, such as reviewing patients on routine medical follow-up, conducting surgical pre-assessments, and undertaking some medical procedures such as endoscopy (Farrell et al. 2011). Whilst such moves created a wealth of opportunities for nurses to expand their current roles or create new ones, it resulted in many nursing roles becoming unrecognisable, with a lack of clarity regarding their roles, responsibilities, and competencies. Amidst this confusion and blurred boundaries with medical colleagues, nurses are trying to find their way to meet new clinical demands whilst meeting patients' needs. It is important that new service developments focus on patient benefits rather than cost savings; however nurses are often caught in the cross-fire. Nurses are clearly embracing the new opportunities and medical responsibilities, and in some cases this means acquiring new technical skills and undertaking medical procedures. However, good communication skills and compassionate care are equally important, and will provide key benefits for patients with improved experiences and clinical outcomes.

Nursing expertise can be linked to a framework of role extension where role expansion and development lie within a continuum (Daly and Carnwell 2003). This is similar to Benner's framework of nursing practice, using five levels from novice to expert (Benner 1984). However, determining the position of individual nurses on a continuum may be problematic, and the phrases of role extension, expansion, and development could become semantics rather than distinct compartments of clinical practice (Callaghan 2007). To understand this further it seems important to consider the concepts, definitions, and clinical aspects of specialist and advanced practice. This will be discussed further in Chapter 3.

Training

Few studies and clinical audits report what training nurses complete in order to undertake their extended role within the nurse-led clinic, which has created uncertainty and disparities in clinical practice. In the UK training includes clinical examination skills (Sheppard et al. 2009, Winter et al. 2011), shadowing or observing doctors (Moore et al. 1999, Sardell et al. 2000, Sheppard et al. 2009), and nonmedical prescribing (Winter et al. 2011). There is evidence in the literature identifying disparate levels of training and lack of clarity in nurses' roles (Torn and McNichol 1998, Lloyd-Jones 2005, Williamson et al. 2012), including results from a survey of oncology-specialist nurses in the UK (Farrell et al. 2011).

Whilst some hospitals in the UK may place mandatory educational requirements for advanced practice roles, including clinical nurse specialist, nurse practitioner, and nurse consultant (Hopwood 2006), this is not a national requirement in the UK. A recent survey identified that clinical skills training for nurse specialists and nurse practitioners was primarily 'in house' and ad hoc, with no formal structure, and similar disparities were evident for nurse consultants, lead nurses, and chemotherapy nurses (Farrell et al. 2011). However, the mandatory requirement for advanced nurse practitioners / nurse clinicians in the UK to undertake clinical skills training within a master's degree in advanced nursing practice provides some standardisation and regulation of roles, although the titles remain unprotected. Evidence in the literature supports the findings that advanced nurse practitioners receive clinical training at master's level (Williamson et al. 2012), whilst training disparities created a lack of role recognition for nurse practitioners (Torn and McNichol 1998). Where clinical examination skills training is not undertaken as part of a university accredited course, there is a lack of standardisation in training and assessments of competency. This is an important issue for nurses since nurses' skills may not be recognised outside their own organisation, which may cause problems when moving to a different hospital trust. Extending nurses' roles in this way also has implications for patients and colleagues, since it creates a lack of clarity and understanding regarding the nurse's role and scope of clinical practice. These issues highlight that greater transparency is needed for advanced nursing practice, including a competency framework for role development, and ongoing training and appraisals of clinical practice.

Whilst one could speculate that monitoring ongoing training is unnecessary since this is not a requirement of medical staff, it does raise concerns if nurses are not using their skills after training, or using them infrequently. This contrasts with intravenous skills training, where there is a more rigorous and clearly defined competency framework for training and ongoing assessments. The introduction of the National Health Service (NHS) Knowledge and Skills Framework (DH 2004) can provide a framework for continuing development (Mills and Pritchard 2004). However, the vast amount of detail within each domain of the framework, the necessity for cross-referencing across the domains, and areas of repetition make this process unwieldy. Furthermore it fails to incorporate some of the complexities within advanced practice roles.

Alternative clinical nursing models

The European Working Time Directive (Goddard et al. 2010, Pickersgill 2001) was one of the main drivers for nurse-led clinics. In addition, alternative clinical nursing models have provided a much needed and welcome breakthrough.

In the 1970s, the concept of the nursing process was introduced in the UK, which was a four-stage model incorporating assessment, planning, implementation, and evaluation (MacFarlane and Castledine 1982). More recently nursing models of care during follow-up after cancer treatment focus on encouraging patient self-management. A systematic review of cancer follow-up suggests the potential benefits of coordinated transition planning, and recommends further research to evaluate the efficacy of models of care (Howell et al. 2012). This has implications for multidisciplinary and also nurse-led care planning, or modelling. However the current lack of theoretical underpinning to clinical models of care needs to be addressed in order to bridge the gap between theory and practice.

Corner (1995) developed an integrative approach to breathlessness, considering the synergistic effect of emotional and physical experiences. This led to the development of a 'parallel model of care', which sits alongside the traditional biomedical model (Krishnasamy et al. 2001). The parallel model is characterised by a requirement to work with the mind and body, and development of a therapeutic relationship with the patient based on partnership and mutual inquiry, which contrasts with the passivity of patients in the biomedical model (Krishnasamy et al. 2001). This model has proved inspirational by identifying different ways of working with a clear application to nurses' clinical practice, focusing on patient benefits and outcomes.

Newton and McVicar (2013) evaluate the currency of the Davies and Oberle (1990) model of supportive care within palliative care. At the centre of this model, preserving one's own integrity related to the nurses' role and the 'respect, authenticity and honesty' of the person, which were regarded as key attributes within palliative care (Simon et al. 2009). The recent evaluation demonstrated that the six dimensions within the model are current and relevant within palliative care: valuing the patient, connecting, empowering, doing for, finding meaning, and preserving one's own integrity. However two new dimensions also emerged: displaying expertise, and influencing other professionals, which reflect current developments in advanced nursing practice and nursing leadership (Newton and McVicar 2013).

Clinical nursing models

A wide variety of models are described within the literature, encompassing a range of meaning from organisational models of service delivery and processes (Dubois et al. 2012), to specific service models of specialist areas such as chronic disease management for epilepsy (Fitzsimmons et al. 2012), or cardiac rehabilitation (Clark et al. 2015). Models also describe aspects of care or consultations, for example integrated care for chronic wounds (Rosenbaum 2012). Therefore the disparate concepts and interpretation of models within the NHS has created great variability in their application, which appears to have diluted the impact on nurses' clinical practice and recognition of changes to nurses' roles.

The lack of theoretical and empirical evidence for changes in organisational models of care has created disparities in clinical service delivery and inconsistent classifications of how nursing care is organised at a unit level (Dubois et al. 2012,

Aiken and Patrician 2000, Jennings 2008). However a conceptual model is considered central to developing service delivery systems by facilitating the identification of systems, processes, and major components, and enabling the analysis of resources and processes in relation to outcomes (McLaughlin and Jordan 2004).

Nurses are involved in all aspects of healthcare delivery across different settings, therefore the way that nursing resources are organised is critical to the organisation's performance; in addition healthcare managers are being challenged to find operational models that maximise available nursing resources (Dubois et al. 2012). Hospitals have had to restructure the way clinical services are delivered in order to meet increasing demand, which has led to a growth in nurse-led models of care. The development of the advanced nurse practitioner has created a hybrid role, bridging the gap between nursing and medicine. However, the emphasis on clinical tasks, such as clinical procedures, clinical examination, and diagnosis appears to have driven a wedge in the identity of nursing, with the greater focus on medical tasks than nursing care.

Given the move towards multidisciplinary working practices, the NHS has introduced the NHS Change Model, which has been created to support the NHS in adopting a shared approach to leading change and transformation (NHS Improving Quality 2013). It includes eight components:

- Our shared purpose
- Leadership for change
- Spread of innovation
- Improvement methodology
- Rigorous delivery
- Transparent measurement
- System drivers
- Engagement to mobilise

The improving capability directorate is working to roll out the NHS Change Model across NHS England as a single approach to transformation and change across the NHS and aims to test its application in different care settings. There are also plans to incorporate the 6Cs (care, compassion, competence, communication, courage, commitment) within this model (NHS Improving Quality 2013).

Legislation and accountability for nurses' roles

All nurses in the UK should be familiar with the NMC Code of Conduct (NMC 2008), which outlines the mandatory requirements of nurses' professional conduct. This includes general principles of behaviour and accountability for nurses within their professional practice, and against which nurses can face disciplinary action. However, in addition nurses should be aware of the legal implications, which have a greater potential impact where nurses extend their roles and take on additional clinical responsibilities that were traditionally undertaken by medical staff.

There are different types of legislation applicable to nurses' roles and responsibilities, including the criminal justice system and the scope or boundaries of professional practice. Certain legislation must be in place before nurses can undertake certain activities that have traditionally been doctors' responsibilities. This section outlines the different types of law relevant to nursing, explaining their meaning in order to understand the implications for clinical practice.

Types of law relevant to nursing

In many countries the scope of nurses' practice is specified in legislation, which includes a definition of nursing and sometimes specific nursing acts. However there is no similar legislation in the UK, although responsibility lies with the profession's regulatory body, the NMC (RCN 2003). In the UK there are several types of legislation applicable to nurses and nurses' roles (see Table 2.1).

Table 2.1 Types of laws relevant to nursing

Type of law	Description
Professional law	Governed by the NMC and code for professional conduct. Focuses on accountability and main ethical principles.
Employment law	Ensures nurses are accountable to their employer, and have a duty to act with reasonable skill and care, obey reasonable orders, maintain confidentiality, and not compete with the employer's business.
	In vicarious liability the employer is held accountable for the 'wrongful acts' of an employee whilst in the course of employment, and is liable to pay damages.
Statute laws	Enacted by the crown in Parliament and provide a broad framework to rules within professional practice: if an advanced nurse practitioner (ANP) takes on a task previously performed by a doctor they must perform it to the same standard as a doctor.
Public law	Governs the Department of Health and NHS, and all employees. If a nurse has broken public law, criminal proceedings would follow in addition to actions by the NMC and the nurse's employer.
Civil law	Refers to actions between individuals and the state. 4 areas will be assessed: • whether there has been a failure in the duty of care • the standard of care • whether there is a causal link between the duty of care and the harm suffered • if harm was a reasonably foreseeable consequence of the breach of duty
Tort law	Enables a patient to bring an action against an ANP for negligence.

Professional law is governed by the NMC, and the code for professional conduct, which focuses on the main ethical principles of autonomy, beneficence, nonmaleficence, and justice (NMC 2008). The NMC Code of Conduct (NMC 2010 p2) states:

> As a professional, you are personally accountable for actions and omissions in your practice, and must always be able to justify your decisions. You must always act lawfully, whether those laws relate to your professional practice or personal life.

In addition to professional accountability with the NMC, nurses have a contractual accountability to their employer and are accountable in law for their actions (NMC 2013).

Statute laws are enacted by the Crown in Parliament and give a broad framework to the rules; if ANPs take on a task previously performed by a doctor they must perform it to the same standard as a doctor (Duke 2012).

Public law governs the Department of Health (DH) and NHS, and all employees. If a nurse has broken public law, criminal proceedings would follow in addition to actions by the NMC and the nurse's employer.

Civil law refers to actions between individuals and the state. *Tort law* enables a patient to bring an action against an ANP for negligence.

Employment law ensures ANPs are accountable to their employer, and have a duty to act with reasonable skill and care, obey reasonable orders, maintain confidentiality, and not compete with the employer's business. In vicarious liability the employer is held accountable for the 'wrongful acts' of an employee whilst in the course of employment, and is liable to pay damages.

The RCN (2012) claims that advanced nurse practitioners carry the same risk of claims of negligence as other nurses, given the educational underpinning to their role. The principle of vicarious liability determines that it is the employer who is sued, rather than an individual nurse, unless the nurse is self-employed (RCN 2012). However, individual nurses at any level must ensure that they work within their own area of competence and knowledge. Legislation has also taken place to enable nurses to prescribe medicines independently, and this will be discussed in Chapter 5.

Summary

Changes to nurses' roles have arisen ad hoc and largely in response to increases in clinical demands, exacerbated by a reduction in junior medical staff. Nurses' willingness to step up to the plate and bridge the gaps in clinical services is commendable and this has created additional opportunities for nurses in a variety of disciplines and specialities. However, the nature of such sporadic changes and lack of consistency locally and nationally has created new challenges. Whilst nurses' individual scope of practice may be determined locally and training/competencies agreed at trust level, this may not be transparent to others, including colleagues and patients. Individual and local variations in nurses' roles and responsibilities, together with a lack of protection for some nurses' titles, have resulted in great disparities in nursing roles across the UK and a lack of transparency. However, in addition to the general irritations that this may cause, it can lead to specific difficulties when nurses want to relocate and their training and skills are neither recognised nor transferable between organisations.

The importance of legislation and accountability when nurses extend their roles should not be underestimated, particularly with advanced nursing practice and where nurses work independently in nurse-led clinics. Whilst support from medical consultants and nurse managers is crucial, well-written protocols for clinical practice and good documentation are vital. We work in a litigious society, therefore we must ensure precise patient records to accurately reflect our clinical practice.

References

Aiken LH, Patrician PA. (2000). Measuring organisational traits of hospitals: the revised nursing work index. *Nursing Research*. 49: 146–153.

Benner P. (1984). *From novice to expert: excellence and power in clinical nursing practice*. Menlo Park, CA, Addison Wesley.

Bryant-Lukosius D, DiCenso A, Browne G, Pinelli J. (2004). Advanced practice nursing roles: development, implementation and evaluation. *Journal of Advanced Nursing*. 48(5): 519–529.

Callaghan L. (2007). Advanced nursing practice: an idea whose time has come. *Journal of Clinical Nursing*. 17: 205–213.

Clark RA, Conway A, Poulson V, Tirimacco R, Tideman P. (2015). Alternative models of cardiac rehabilitation. *European Journal of Preventative Cardiology*. 22 (1): 35–74.

Corner J. (1995). Innovative approaches in symptom management. *European Journal of Cancer Care*. 4: 145–146.

Daly WM, Carnwell R. (2003). Nursing roles and levels of practice: a framework for differentiating between elementary, specialist and advanced nursing practice. *Journal of Nursing Practice*. 12: 158–170.

Davies B, Oberle K. (1990). Dimensions of the supportive role of the nurse in palliative care. *Oncology Nursing Forum*. 17: 87–93.

Department of Health. (2004). NHS Knowledge and Skills Framework (KSF). London, DH.

Dubois CA, D'Amour D, Tchouaket E, Rivard M, Clarke S, Blais R. (2012). A taxonomy of nursing care organization models in hospitals. *BMC Health Service Research*. 12: 286–301.

Duke N. (2012). Exploring advanced nursing practice: past, present and future. *British Journal of Nursing*. 21(17): 26–30.

Farrell C. (2014). *An exploration of oncology nurse specialists' roles in nurse-led chemotherapy clinics*. Unpublished PhD thesis, University of Manchester.

Farrell C, Molassiotis A, Beaver K, Heaven C. (2011). Exploring the scope of oncology specialist nurses' practice in the UK. *European Journal of Oncology Nursing*. 15(2): 160–166.

Fitzsimmons M, Normand C, Varley J, Delanty N. (2012). Evidence-based models of care for people with epilepsy. *Epilepsy Behaviour*. 23(1): 1–6.

Folland S. (2000). Redefining the role of the clinical nurse specialist. *European Journal of Palliative Care*. 7(5): 172–174.

Gardner G, Chang A, Duffield C. (2007). Making nursing work: breaking through the role confusion of advanced practice nursing. *Journal of Advanced Nursing*. 57 (4): 382–391.

Goddard A, Hodgson H, Newbery N. (2010). Impact of EWTD on patient: doctor rations and working practices for junior doctors in England and Wales. *Clinical Medicine*. 10(4): 1–6.

Henderson V. (2006). The concept of nursing. *Journal of Advanced Nursing*. 53(1): 21–34.

Hopwood L. (2006). Developing advanced nursing practice roles in cancer care. *Nursing Times*. 102(15): 40–41.

Howell D, Hack TF, Oliver TK, Chulak T, Mayo S, Aubin M, Chasen M, Earle CC, Friedman AJ, Green E, Jones GW, Jones JM, Parkinson M, Payeur N, Sabiston CM, Sinclair S. (2012). Models of care for post-treatment follow-up of adult cancer survivors: a systematic review and quality appraisal of the evidence. *Journal of Cancer Survivorship*. 6(4): 359–371.

Jennings BM. (2008). Care models. In: *Patient safety and quality: an evidence-based handbook for nurses*. Edited by Hughes RG. Rockville MD: Agency for Healthcare Research and Quality. 1–10.

Krishnasamy M, Corner J, Bredin M, Plant H, Bailey C. (2001). Cancer nursing practice development: understanding breathlessness. *Journal of Clinical Nursing*. 10: 103–108.

Lloyd-Jones M. (2005). Role development and effective practice in specialist and advanced practice roles in acute hospital settings: systematic review and meta-analysis. *Journal of Advanced Nursing*. 49(2): 191–209.

Mills C, Pritchard T. (2004). A competency framework for nurses in specialist roles. *Nursing Times*. 100(43): 28–29.

Moore S, Corner J, Fuller F. (1999). Development of nurse-led follow up in the management of patients with lung cancer. *Nursing Times Research*. 4: 432–444.

MacFarlane J, Castledine G. (1982). *A guide to the practice of nursing: Using the nursing process*. London, CV Moseby.

McLaughlin J, Jordan GB. (2004). Handbook of practical programme evaluation. In: *Using logic models*, 2nd ed. Edited by Wholey J, Hatry HP, Newcomer KE. San Francisco, Jossey-Bass. 7–32.

Newton J and McVicar A. (2013). An evaluation of the currency of the Davies and Oberle (1990) model of supportive care in specialist and specialised palliative care settings in England. *Journal of Clinical Nursing*. 23(11–12): 1662–1676.

NHS Improving Quality. (2013). *The NHS change model*. http://www.nhsiq.nhs.uk/capacity-capability/nhs-change-model.aspx [accessed 19.10.2013].

Nursing and Midwifery Council. (2008). *The code: standards of conduct, performance and ethics for nurses and midwives*. London. NMC.

Nursing and Midwifery Council. (2010). *The proposed framework for the standard for post registration nursing*. http://www.nmc-uk.org/Get-involved/Consultations/Past-consultations/By-year/The-proposed-framework-for-the-standard-for-post-registration-nursing-February-2005/ [accessed 19.10.2013].

Nursing and Midwifery Council. (2013). *Regulation in practice*. http://www.nmc-uk.org/Nurses-and-midwives/Regulation-in-practice/ [accessed 19.10.2013].

Pickersgill T. (2001). The European working time directive for doctors in training. *British Medical Journal*. 323: 1266.

RCN Competencies. (2012). *Advanced nurse practitioners: an RCN guide to advanced nursing practice, advanced nurse practitioners and programme accreditation.* London, Royal College of Nursing.

Royal College of Nursing. (2003). *Defining nursing.* London. RCN.

Rosenbaum C. (2012). An overview of integrative care options for patients with chronic wounds. *Ostomy Wound Management.* 58(5): 44–51.

Sardell S, Sharpe G, Ashley S, Guerrero D, Brada M. (2000). Evaluation of a nurse-led telephone clinic in the follow up of patients with malignant glioma. *Clinical Oncology.* 12(1): 36–41.

Sheppard C, Higgins B, Wise M, Yiangou C, Dubois D, Kilburn S. (2009). Breast cancer follow up: a randomised controlled trial comparing point of need access versus routine 6-monthly clinical review. *European Journal of Oncology Nursing.* 13: 2–8.

Simon ST, Ramsenthaler C, Bausewein C, Krischke N, Geiss G. (2009). Core attitudes of professionals in palliative care: a qualitative study. *International Journal of Palliative Nursing.* 15: 405–411.

Torn A, McNichol, E. (1998). A qualitative study utilizing focus group to explore the role and concept of the nurse practitioner. *Journal of Advanced Nursing.* 27: 1202–1211.

UKCC. (1992). *The scope of professional practice.* London, UKCC.

Williamson S, Twelvetree T, Thompson J, Beaver K. (2012). An ethnographic study exploring the role of ward-based advanced nurse practitioners in an acute medical setting. *Journal of Advanced Nursing.* 68(7): 1579–1588.

Winter H, Lavender V, Blesing C. (2011). Developing a nurse-led clinic for patients enrolled in clinical trials. *Cancer Nursing Practice.* 10(3): 20–24.

Chapter 3

Advanced nursing practice and clinical leadership

Carole Farrell

This chapter seeks to define advanced nursing practice, discussing key components, skills, and competencies. This will form a framework for advanced nursing practice in oncology, and include examples from clinical practice to demonstrate the differences between advanced nursing practice and other levels of clinical practice. Clinical leadership will be outlined, discussing implications for advanced nursing practice.

Specialist practice

Specialist nurses are dedicated to caring for people with long-term conditions and diseases such as cancer, diabetes, Parkinson's disease, chronic heart failure, and dementia (RCN 2010b). Specialist nurses have extensive experience and knowledge within their field of practice, where they are generally seen as expert practitioners (Knowles 2007), however their role does not automatically equate to an advanced level of practice nor automatically result in them becoming an advanced nurse practitioner. The criteria for advanced nursing practice must be considered separately.

Advanced practice

The term *advanced nursing practice* first appeared in the nursing literature in the 1980s (Ruel and Motyka 2009). However many titles, such as nurse practitioner (NP), clinical nurse specialist (CNS), nurse consultant (NC), and nurse clinician, are being adopted in different care settings and various countries, with little understanding of the nature of roles and differences between them, therefore there is little consensus (Daly and Carnwell 2003). The term *advanced practice nurse* or *advanced nurse practitioner* (ANP) is often used within the literature as an all-encompassing term to include various advanced practice titles (Ketefian et al. 2001).

Discrepancies with nursing titles

A systematic review identified that internationally nurses may be working at similar levels of advanced practice although their titles may be dissimilar (Jokiniemi et al. 2012).

In the UK the introduction of the nurse consultant role began in 2000, aiming to improve patient outcomes by improving the quality of clinical services, strengthening nursing leadership, and providing greater career opportunities for clinical nurses (Health Service Circular 1999/217). It was envisaged that nurse consultants would spend at least 50 per cent of their time on direct clinical care with patients or communities; other key areas of practice would include professional leadership and consultancy, research/evaluation, education/training, and service development (Health Service Circular 1999/217).

In the USA, the role of CNS dates back to the early 1940s, defined as an advanced practice nurse with a wide range of theoretical and evidence-based knowledge and educated to master's or doctoral level (Lewandowski & Adamle 2009).

In Australia, the clinical nurse consultant (CNC) was introduced in the mid-1980s (O'Baugh et al. 2007, O'Connor and Chapman 2008), defined as a registered nurse with at least five years post-basic registration experience, and a post-basic nursing qualification relevant to their field of practice (NSW Department of Health 2005).

Such disparities reflect the international lack of consensus on nurses' titles and roles within advanced nursing practice. Jokiniemi et al. (2012) suggest that the common feature in international literature on advanced practice nursing and its subroles is ambiguity.

However, McFadden and Miller (1994) argue that the vague definition of the ANP role may facilitate role development in self-directed individuals, since this enables nurses to define their own priorities in different domains. Nevertheless the current disparities in titles, definitions, and scope of practice have created such confusion amongst nurses, other health professionals, and patients that many suggest some level of standardisation is required (Ketefian et al. 2001, Daly and Carnwell 2003, Glover et al. 2006, Humphreys et al. 2007, Mantzoukas and Watkinson 2007, Lewandowski and Adamle 2009, Farrell et al. 2011). Ruel and Motyka (2009) also claim that a cohesive vision of advanced nursing practice is essential to achieve the external legitimacy that is required to reinforce the need for ANP amongst society, legislators, and stakeholders.

Defining advanced nursing practice

There are many definitions of advanced nursing practice, and the main ones will be outlined in this chapter to discuss the key issues and implications. The RCN (2008) defines an advanced nurse practitioner as a registered nurse with at least a first honours degree. However they also identify a list of 11 essential components of the role, which include making professionally autonomous decisions, for which he/she is accountable, undertaking physical examination, differential diagnosis, ordering investigations, counselling and health education, and leadership (RCN 2008). Following on from this, the RCN go on to define advanced practice as a level of practice rather than a person's role or job title (RCN 2010, 2012b), which reflects the Nursing and Midwifery Council (NMC) definition of advanced nurse practitioners:

> Highly experienced and educated members of the care team who are able to diagnose and treat [patients'] healthcare needs or refer [patients] to an appropriate specialist if needed.
>
> (NHS 2008, 35)

Using these definitions, an ANP in primary care is a generalist, providing complete episodes of care for patients with a wide variety of health needs and problems, or specific illnesses such as depression or heart failure, however works at an advanced level of practice (RCN 2012). An ANP in oncology is a specialist who may provide complete episodes of care for patients within one cancer group, or treatment modality such as chemotherapy.

Exploring advanced nursing practice

The Department of Health report that confusion about the scope of nurses' roles and competence results from 'advanced practice' being inconsistently applied to nurses' roles (DH 2010). However, the NMC (2012) has outlined that advanced nursing practice is an umbrella term to describe a number of specialist roles, which include specialist nurses and advanced nurse practitioners. Although this is a good general explanation, it does little to eradicate the difficulties and challenges that have arisen from a lack of clear definition to guide clinical staff and others working within the NHS.

However, the situation in the UK contrasts with the US, where legislation and regulatory mechanisms provide protected titles for clinical nurse specialists and nurse practitioners (Bryant-Lukosius et al. 2004). Pulcini et al. (2010) identified that 23 out of 32 countries reviewed had formal recognition of nurse practitioner and advanced nurse practitioner roles, and half of them required practitioners to undertake continued practice development in order to maintain or renew their licence.

Specialist and advanced nursing practice

The RCN highlights that a number of nurses are using the title of nurse practitioner and advanced nurse practitioner without undertaking an appropriate level of education or training (RCN 2008). The NMC (2007) describes this as a major concern since it creates a lack of transparency for patients and the general. A position statement from the Department of Health (2010c) also recognises that 'advanced level practice' has been applied inconsistently to a number of different roles, which has often created confusion about the scope and competence required at this level of practice (DH 2010c). Whilst all this mirrors what clinical nurses have been saying for years, and highlights the difficult situation within advanced nursing practice, it seems that little is being done nationally to address these issues at ground level; however guidelines and frameworks for advanced practice are achieving some consensus.

In a position statement the Department of Health (DH 2010c) emphasise that whilst there may be differences in advanced practice roles, it is important that organisations conduct a job evaluation exercise during the post-development process in order to ensure consistency, either by job matching with an existing national profile or through local evaluation systems. The position statement (DH 2010c) provides a benchmark for advanced practice, consisting of 28 elements across four themes:

- Clinical/direct care practice
- Leadership and collaborative practice
- Improving quality and developing practice
- Developing self and others

Nurses working at an advanced level are described as practice leaders, managing their own workload and working across professional, organisational, agency, and system boundaries in order to improve clinical services and develop nursing practice, whilst networking locally and nationally (DH 2010). In addition, nurses in advanced practice often have a track record of innovative practice and service development, such as leading/designing and delivering new care pathways and services; and developing and implementing policy, standards, guidelines, and protocols (DH 2010c).

UK frameworks for advanced nursing practice

Scotland developed a framework for specialist and advanced practice which builds on the core-level capability framework for nurses and allied health professionals (NES 2007). This was based on the Skills for Health (2006) framework, consisting of nine levels of practice. Within the nine levels, levels one through four represent healthcare support workers and assistant practitioners, whilst levels five through nine represent registered nurses (see Table 3.1) (NES 2008). This provides clear distinctions between specialist and advanced practice, incorporating senior roles such as nurse consultants.

NES (2007a) identifies four themes for advanced practice: leadership, facilitating learning, research, advanced clinical practice. The themes are underpinned by several key principles which should be evidenced by all nurses working at an advanced level:

- Autonomous practice
- Critical thinking

Table 3.1 Scottish framework for advanced practice (Skills for Health 2006)

Level of practice	Generic title	Description
Level 5	Practitioner	Registered practitioners in their first and second post-registration / professional qualification job
Level 6	Senior or specialist practitioner	Staff with a higher degree of autonomy and responsibility than practitioners in the clinical environment
Level 7	Advanced practitioner	Experienced clinical staff with a very high standard of skills and theoretical knowledge, making high-level clinical decisions and often having their own caseload
Level 8	Consultant practitioner	Staff working at a very high level of clinical expertise and / or have responsibility for planning services
Level 9	More senior staff	Staff with the ultimate responsibility for clinical decision-making and full on-call accountability

- High levels of decision-making and problem-solving skills
- Values-based-care
- Improving practice (NES 2008)

Wilson and Holt (2001) argue that competencies do not take into account the complexities within clinical practice. However, capability describes the extent to which an individual can apply, adapt and synthesise new knowledge and continue to improve their performance (Fraser and Greenhalgh 2001), which is essential for effective practitioners (NES 2008). This reflects Benner's definitions of an expert practitioner who is able to adapt in unpredictable and unfamiliar circumstances (Benner 1984).

The knowledge and skills framework (KSF)

The NES (2007, 2008) also introduced templates using the KSF to demonstrate consistency across common elements linked to advanced practice, which can be used to determine post outlines (see Table 3.2)

In 2009 NHS Wales accepted the principles within the Scottish Government Health Department's Advanced Practice Toolkit (SGHD 2008), which was developed by Scotland on behalf of the other three home nations and combines UK and International work on advanced level practice. The Toolkit demonstrates consensus on advanced levels of practice and provides tools and resources to support the implementation of roles (www.advancedpractice.scot.nhs.uk).

Table 3.2 Incorporating KSF into advanced practice roles

KSF Core dimension	Nature of dimension	Competency level	Domains of advanced practice
Dimension I	Communication	Level 4	Clinical, management, leadership, education
Dimension 2	Personal and people development	Level 4	Management, leadership, education
Dimension 3	Quality	Level 3	Clinical, research
Dimension 4	Health and well-being dimensions	Level 4	Clinical

The Scottish advanced practice toolkit

The Scottish advanced practice toolkit is web-based and contains a number of very useful tools and resources, including:

*   A competency map / competency assessment guidance
*   A national Agenda for Change (AfC) job profile for advanced practice, KSF outlines, and job descriptions / role profiles
*   Activity analysis / skills analysis / educational needs analysis tools
*   Mapping of education programme outcomes to competencies and capabilities
*   Regulatory guidance (SGHD 2008)

NES (2007) also identifies four 'pillars' of advanced practice, which signify broad areas or domains of practice:

1. Management and leadership
2. Education
3. Research
4. Advanced clinical practice

In addition, key factors for nurse consultants are identified that may be used to distinguish between advanced practice and consultant levels of practice (NES 2008):

*   High levels of strategic thinking, knowledge, and skills, commensurate with expert practice
*   Roles accountable preferably at board level, and senior management level as a minimum
*   Undertaking and integrating research into clinical practice
*   Working strategically across a range of models of service delivery
*   Influencing policy and decision-making (NES 2008)

Mills and Pritchard (2004) suggest that advanced nursing practice focuses on how and what nurses do, rather than their qualifications, and therefore places greater emphasis on competencies within clinical practice. Distinguishing between advanced practice and nurse consultant levels, the National Leadership and Innovation Agency for Healthcare (NLIAH 2011) suggest that nurse consultants have higher levels of strategic thinking, knowledge, and skills, integrate research into clinical practice, and work strategically across a range of models of service delivery (NLIAH 2011).

In a systematic review of advanced practice roles in the UK, USA, and Australia, the roles of the nurse consultant, clinical nurse specialist, and clinical nurse consultant were found to be similar, however variation appeared to come from organisational or individual choices, rather than individual countries (Jokiniemi et al. 2012). Role domains identified were advanced clinical practice, practice development, education, research, consultation, and administration (Jokiniemi et al. 2012).

In other studies, advanced clinical practice appeared to be the central domain (Vaughan et al. 2005, Jinks and Chalder 2007, Redwood et al. 2007) accounting for 23 to 50 per cent of the advanced practice nurse's total working time (Charters et al. 2005, Darmody 2005, Jinks & Chalder 2007). However, a reduction in the expert clinical practice of nurse consultants was noticed over time, with a shift towards more strategic engagement within acute care trusts (Dawson and Coombs 2008). In the UK there are similar disparities within several oncology specialist nurses' roles, including nurse consultants, nurse practitioners, and clinical nurse specialists, suggesting individual and local influences on what nurses do within their role (Farrell et al. 2011).

Clinical skills

Advancements in clinical examination skills have become synonymous with advanced nursing practice, as though a nurse can only be seen as an advanced practitioner if he or she uses a stethoscope. Again this places emphasis on doctor-nurse substitution and medical models of care. In reality there are disparities in nurses' clinical skills, including clinical examination skills, with significant differences in groups of nurses who undertook respiratory and abdominal examinations (Farrell 2014). Comparing NCs, ANPs, NPs, LNs, and CNSs, advanced nurse practitioners undertook the most extensive range of clinical examinations, whilst there was variability across the other groups; although nurse practitioners all undertook local clinical examinations, they did not perform any cardiovascular or top to toe examinations, and only one conducted respiratory examinations (Farrell 2014) (see Figure 3.1)

Nurses in the survey also reported a wide variety of other medical assessments, which included surgical pre assessments, wound checks, and disease-specific procedures and medical investigations. Those conducted by clinical nurse specialists' included practical skills, such as blood tests and seroma assessments, but

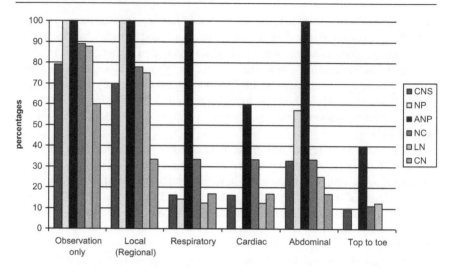

Figure 3.1 Range of clinical examinations across groups of nurses

also more advanced medical investigations, for example colposcopies and biopsies. In addition, some CNSs conducted family history screening/assessment and formulated clinical management plans. In comparison, nurse practitioners were mainly involved in booking scans, ordering pathology, draining seromas, and assessing wounds. In contrast, advanced nurse practitioners did not seem to be as task-orientated as the clinical nurse specialists and nurse practitioners. Their role focused on assessment, screening and diagnosis, assessing possible relapse, and monitoring late effects of treatment. Nurse consultants reported undertaking 'out of hours' telephone advice, family history screening/assessment, and biopsies. Some nurses undertook more specific aspects of clinical management, such as lymphoedema, counselling, and pain management. Lead nurses appeared to have similar responsibilities to advanced practitioners in detecting disease progression, requesting and reviewing bloods and imaging, and making referrals to colleagues as necessary (Farrell 2014).

Valuing nurses' roles

A national survey of health advocacy groups identified that patients rated specialist nurses higher than any other health professional in understanding patient needs, designing and implementing care pathways, obtaining patient feedback, and being transparent and honest (RCN 2008). However, a survey of specialist nurses in 2005/6 showed that one in four specialist nurses faced redundancy, half were aware of service cuts in their speciality, and 45 per cent were being asked to work outside their speciality to cover staff shortages elsewhere (RCN 2008). In addition 47 per cent of specialist nurses reported that they were at risk of being downgraded, and 68 per cent reported having to see more patients (RCN 2008). There are also reports that nearly one in four specialist nurses faced risk of redundancy and many were asked to fill vacancies and shortages in other settings within the NHS (RCN 2013, 2010). However there is also clear evidence demonstrating that specialist nurses can improve the lives of their patients and deliver value for money (Macmillan 2011, Williams 2011, RCN 2012a, Price 2012). This highlights current tensions within the NHS.

In a recent survey the majority of nurses perceived their role was highly valued (n=44, 55.7%) within the multidisciplinary team (MDT); however 11 (13.9%) felt their role was occasionally valued and one nurse felt that their role was not valued at all (Farrell 2014). This is reflected in nurses' comments:

'MDT are appreciative of CNS role – much of our extended roles has reduced clinician workload . . .' [CNS]

This is reflected in other groups of nurses:

'Within the MDT / care team. The role is valued for its leadership, service development, strategic direction, consultancy role' [NC]
'Especially when medical cover needed' [ANP]

However some nurses suggest that perceptions about their roles have changed over time, and are no longer feel valued:

'I think it was highly valued at first but now I fear it's invisible' [CNS]
'I am repeatedly told I am an expensive nurse who needs to prove my worth' [CNS]

(Farrell 2014, 144)

Although research is considered important for advanced practice roles, involvement in research remains generally low (Jokinicmi et al. 2012, Farrell et al. 2011), and lack of time was the main factor cited for this (Dawson and McEwen 2005, Farrell et al. 2011).

Organisational challenges, including lack of managerial support, were found to aggravate the implementation of advanced practice roles (Jokiniemi et al. 2012, Farrell et al. 2011), exacerbated by vague definitions and role ambiguity (Abbott 2007, Charters et al. 2005, Redwood et al. 2007, O'Connor and Chapman 2008).

From novice to expert practice

There has also been considerable debate regarding specialist practice, and its position in relation to the development of advanced practice. Some nurses appear to

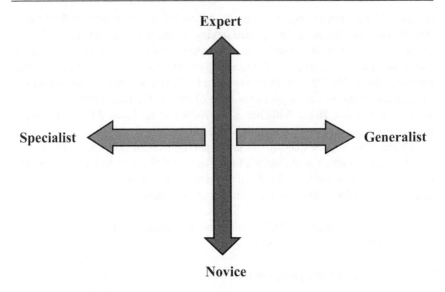

Figure 3.2 Relationship between specialist and advanced practice

Source: Adapted from NLIAH 2011

have a misconception that specialist nursing is a higher level than general nursing, and that advanced nursing practice is a higher level of practice than specialist nursing. This seems based on an assumption (made incorrectly) that there is one continuum of development for nurses through clinical practice, incorporating general, specialist, and advanced practice. However, there is increasing acceptance that specialist practice should be considered as one pole on the continuum of specialist and generalist, and a separate development continuum from novice to expert (NLIAH 2011) (see Figure 3.2).

At some point, for each individual, the two lines will intersect, which will show:

1. Where a nurse's role lies on the continuum from generalist to specialist practice
2. Where a nurse's role lies on the development continuum from novice to expert

Consequently a nurse may be regarded as a novice generalist or novice specialist, an advanced generalist or advanced specialist, including different stages between these extremes (NLIAH 2011). Using this model, the continuum of novice to expert reflects nurses' level of clinical practice and competencies; in contrast the generalist-to-specialist continuum is descriptive, indicating the nature of nurses' area of practice.

This overview crosses all domains of nursing, placing emphasis on the level of nurses' practice and developments towards advanced clinical practice, rather than descriptors such as nurses' titles or areas of clinical practice.

Advanced practice should be seen as a stage on the continuum from novice to expert, characterised by high levels of clinical skills, competence, and autonomous decision-making (NLIAH 2011). Therefore, within a specialist area there will be nurses working at different levels of practice from novice to advanced; specialist nurses are specialists within one specific area of practice, which may include caring for people with long-term conditions and diseases such as cancer, diabetes, Parkinson's disease, chronic heart failure, and dementia (RCN 2010). In oncology, the title CNS is generally used to describe a skilled practitioner with expert knowledge working at an advanced level in a specialist area (Knowles 2007). The presumption that specialist nurses are all working at an advanced level seems erroneous and misleading.

Influences on nurses' roles and advanced practice

Pulcini et al. (2010) report that support for advanced nursing roles came from domestic nursing organisations (92%), individual nurses (70%), and government (68%); whilst opposition to introducing advanced nursing roles came primarily from doctors (83%) and doctor organisations (67%) (Pulcini et al. 2010). This highlights tensions between medicine and nursing in relation to the expansion of nurses' roles and reflects comments from nurses in other countries regarding such challenges. In some cases this appears to be driven by monetary gain within private health services overseas. However, there are also examples within the UK of power tensions between medical consultants and nurses in relation to nurse-led clinics, illustrating the control doctors can exert to influence the scope of nurses' clinical practice and their nurse-led clinics (Farrell 2014).

Thorpe (1997) reports that some nurse practitioners have been employed specifically to undertake medical tasks, such as admitting and clerking patients, which may restrict a nursing focus of care. An ethnographic study of advanced nurse practitioners on hospital wards identified that other nurses perceived their roles to be more closely allied with medicine than nursing, although they were viewed as more approachable than doctors and had a positive impact on nursing practice (Williamson et al. 2012). In contrast, an ethnographic study of nurse-led chemotherapy clinics identified disparities between nurses' perceptions of their roles and behaviour / communication skills, in that nurses emphasised the importance of being a nurse and undertaking holistic assessments, yet in many cases this was not apparent during observations of their clinical consultations, where nurses tended to use a medical model (Farrell 2014).

Summary

Despite the advances in nursing practice and improvements in nursing legislation to support it, there is a current lack of clarity regarding competencies for advanced practice and no clear role definition for advanced nurse practitioners. This is exacerbated given the plethora of nursing titles and lack of clear definition and regulation for the use of new titles, such as nurse practitioner and advanced nurse practitioner, which may cause confusion for patients, the public, and other health-care professionals. From this it seems important to undertake further research to explore more fully the concept of advanced nursing practice and new roles within it.

There is some evidence in the literature highlighting how nurses' roles are changing and the impact this may have on others. An ethnographic study of advanced nurse practitioners highlights their role in teaching junior medical and nursing staff, which is seen to promote advanced nurse practitioners as role models for both professions (Williamson et al. 2012). However, this also shows how the role of advanced nurse practitioners may de-skill ward nurses by reducing their use of analytical skills, particularly when time is limited (Williamson et al. 2012).

Managers may also face difficulties when nurses expand their existing role if nurses' scope of practice and job description is not well defined (Torn and McNichol 1998); therefore clear lines of communication seem vital. Furthermore, since the majority of new cancer nursing roles have developed with little evidence of evaluation, it seems difficult to appreciate their impact and effectiveness on patients and cancer service delivery, and this may lead hospital managers to question their value.

References

Abbott S. (2007). Leadership across boundaries: a qualitative study of the nurse consultant role in English primary care. *Journal of Nursing Management*. 15: 703–710.

Benner PA. (1984). *From novice to expert: excellence and power in clinical nursing practice*. Menlo Park, CA, Addison Wesley.

Bryant-Lukosius D, DiCenso A, Browne G, Pinelli J. (2004). Advanced practice nursing roles: development, implementation and evaluation. *Journal of Advanced Nursing*. 48(5): 519–529.

Charters S, Knight S, Currie J, Davies-Gray M, Ainsworth-Smith M, Smith S, Crouch R. (2005). Learning from the past to inform the future – a survey of consultant nurses in emergency care. *Accident and Emergency Nursing*. 13: 186–193.

Darmody JV. (2005). Observing the work of the clinical nurse specialist: a pilot study. *Clinical Nurse Specialist*. 19: 260–268.

Daly WM, Carnwell R. (2003). Nursing roles and levels of practice: a framework for differentiating between elementary, specialist and advancing nursing practice. *J. Clin. Nurs.* 12: 158–167.

Dawson D, Coombs M. (2008). The current role of the consultant nurse in critical care: consolidation or consternation? *Intensive Critical Care Nursing*. 24: 187–196.

Dawson D, McEwen A. (2005). Critical care without walls: the role of the nurse consultant in critical care. *Intensive Critical Care Nursing*. 21: 334–343.

Department of Health. (2010c). *Advanced nursing practice: a position statement*. London, DH.

Farrell C. (2014). *An exploration of oncology nurse specialists' roles in nurse-led chemotherapy clinics*. Unpublished PhD thesis, University of Manchester.

Farrell C, Molassiotis A, Beaver K, Heaven C. (2011). Exploring the scope of oncology specialist nurses' practice in the UK. *European Journal of Oncology Nursing.* 15(2): 160–166.

Fraser SW, Greenhalgh T. (2001). Coping with complexity: educating for capability. *British Medical Journal.* 323: 799–803.

Glover DE, Newkirk LE, Cole LM, Walker TJ, Nader KC. (2006). Perioperative clinical nurse specialist role delineation: a systematic review. *AORN J.* 84: 1017–1030.

Health Service Circular. (1999). *Nurse, midwife and health visitor consultants. Establishing posts and making appointments.* Series Number: HSC 1999/217. Available at http://www.dh.gov.uk/prod_consum_dh/groups/dh_digitalassets/@dh/@en/documents/digitalasset/dh_4012227.pdf [accessed 23.05.2015].

Humphreys A, Johnson S, Richardson J, Stenhouse E, Watkins M. (2007). A systematic review and meta-synthesis: evaluating the effectiveness of nurse, midwife/allied health professional consultants. *Journal of Clinical Nursing.* 16: 1792–1808.

Jinks A, Chalder G. (2007). Consensus and diversity: an action research study designed to analyze the roles of a group of mental health nurse consultants. *Journal of Clinical Nursing.* 16: 1323–1332.

Jokiniemi K, Pietilä AM, Kylmä J, Haatainen K. (2012). Advanced nursing roles: a systematic review. *Nursing Health Science.* 14(3): 421–31. doi: 10.1111/j.1442-2018.2012.00704.x.

Ketefian S, Redman RW, Hanucharurnkul S, Masterson A, Neves EP. (2001). The development of advanced practice roles: implications in the international nursing community. *Int. Nurs. Rev.* 4: 152–163.

Knowles G. (2007). *Advanced nursing practice framework – Cancer nurse specialist example.* Report prepared for the Scottish Government. Available at http://www.advancedpractice. scot.nhs.uk/media/1282/appendix_1a__1.the_toolkit_concept__1.1overview.pdf [accessed 23.05.2015].

Lewandowski W, Adamle K. (2009). Substantive areas of clinical nurse specialist practice: a comprehensive review of the literature. *Clin. Nurse Spec.* 23: 73–92.

MacMillan Cancer Support. (2011). *Cancer clinical nurse specialists: an evidence review.* Available at http://www.macmillan.org.uk/Documents/AboutUs/Commissioners/Clinic alNurseSpecialistsAnEvidenceReview2011.pdf [accessed 23.05.2015].

Mantzoukas S, Watkinson S. (2007). Review of advanced nursing practice: the international literature and developing the generic features. *Journal of Clinical Nursing.* 16: 28–37.

McFadden EA, Miller MA. (1994). Clinical nurse specialist practice: facilitators and barriers. *Clinical Nurse Specialist.* 8: 27–33.

Mills, C; Pritchard, T. (2004). A competency framework for nurses in specialist roles. *Nursing Times.* 100(43): 28–29.

NHS Education for Scotland. (2007). *Working with individuals with cancer, their families and carers. Professional development framework for nurses and allied health professionals. Core level.* Edinburgh, NES.

NHS Education for Scotland. (2007a). *Advance practice succession planning pathway.* Edinburgh. Edinburgh, NES.

NHS Education for Scotland. (2008). Working with individuals with cancer, their families and carers: Professional development framework for nurses, specialist and advanced levels. Edinburgh, NHS Education for Scotland.

National Leadership and Innovation Agency for Healthcare. (2011). *Framework for advanced nursing, midwifery and allied health professional practice in Wales.* Llanharan, Wales, NLIAH.

Nursing and Midwifery Council, (2005). *Consultation on a framework for the standard for post-registration nursing*. London, NMC.

Nursing and Midwifery Council. (2007). *Advancing nursing practice – update 19 June 2007*. London. NMC. Available at www.nmc-uk.org/aArticle.aspx?ArticleID=2528 [accessed 22.10.2007].

Nursing and Midwifery Council (2012). *Policy areas: advanced nursing practice*. London, NMC.

NSW Department of Health. (2005). *Public health system nurses' and midwives' (state) award – New Award*. Available at http://www.health.nsw.gov.au/policies/ib/2005/pdf/IB2005_063.pdf [accessed 23.05.2015].

O'Baugh J, Wilkes LM, Vaughan K, O'Donohue R. (2007). The role and scope of the clinical nurse consultant in Wentworth Area Health Service, New South Wales, Australia. *Journal of Nursing Management*. 15: 12–21.

O'Connor M, Chapman Y. (2008). The palliative care clinical nurse consultant as an essential link. *Collegian*. 15: 151–157.

Price A. (2012). Specialist nurses improve outcomes in heart failure patients. *Nursing Times*. 108: 40, 22–24.

Pulcini J, Jelic M, Gul R, Loke, AY. (2010). An international survey on advanced practice nursing education, practice, and regulation. *Journal of Nursing Scholarship*. 42(1): 31–39.

RCN. (2008). *Local healthcare commissioning: grassroots involvement: A national survey of health advocacy models*. London, RCN and National Voices.

RCN. (2010). *Advanced nurse practitioners: An RCN guide to advanced nursing practice, advanced nurse practitioners and programme accreditation*. London, RCN.

RCN. (2010b). *Specialist nurses: changing lives, saving money*. Available at http://www.rcn.org.uk/__data/assets/pdf_file/0008/302489/003581.pdf [accessed 23.05.2015].

RCN. (2012a). *Clinical nurse specialist: adding value to care*. Available at http://www.rcn.org.uk/__data/assets/pdf_file/0008/317780/003598.pdf [accessed 23.05.2015].

RCN. (2013). *RCN factsheet: Specialist nursing in the UK*. Available at http://www.rcn.org.uk/__data/assets/pdf_file/0018/501921/4.13_RCN_Factsheet_on_Specialist_nursing_in_UK_-_2013.pdf [accessed 23.05.2015].

RCN Competencies. (2012b). *Advanced nurse practitioners: An RCN guide to advanced nursing practice, advanced nurse practitioners and programme accreditation*. London, RCN.

Redwood S, Lloyd H, Carr E, et al. (2007). Evaluating nurse consultants' work through key informant perceptions. *Nursing Standard*. 21: 35–40.

Ruel J, Motyka C. (2009). Advanced practice nursing: a principle-based concept analysis. *J. Am. Acad. Nurse Pract*. 21: 384–392.

Scottish Government Health Departments. (2008). *Supporting the development of advanced nursing practice – a toolkit approach*. Available at http://www.aanpe.org/LinkClick.aspx?fileticket=giFsLijsCRw%3D&tabid=1051&mid=2508&language=en-US [accessed 23.05.2015].

Skills for Health. (2006). *Career framework for health*. Available at www.skillsforhealth.org.uk/page/career-frameworks [accessed 09.10.2013].

Thorpe P. (1997). Worrying wedge. *Nursing Standard*. 11: 17.

Torn A, McNichol E. (1998). A qualitative study utilizing focus group to explore the role and concept of the nurse practitioner. *Journal of Advanced Nursing*. 27: 1202–1211.

Vaughan K, Wilkes LM, O'Baugh J, O'Donohue R. (2005). The role and scope of the Clinical Nurse Consultant in Wentworth Area Health Service: a qualitative study. *Collegian*. 12: 14–19.

Williams D. (2011). Specialist nurses boost care for lung cancer patients. *Nursing Times*. Available at http://www.nursingtimes.net/nursing-practice/clinical-zones/cancer/specialist-nurses-boost-care-for-lung-cancer-patients/5030101.article [accessed 23. 05.2015].

Williamson S, Twelvetree T, Thompson J, Beaver K. (2012). An ethnographic study exploring the role of ward-based advanced nurse practitioners in an acute medical setting. *Journal of Advanced Nursing*. 68(7): 1579–1588.

Wilson T, Holt T. (2001). Complexity and clinical care. *British Medical Journal*. 323: 685–688.

Chapter 4

Autonomy

Implications for oncology nursing

Carole Farrell

Beginning with definitions of autonomy, this chapter will help to clarify the meaning of autonomy in relation to nurses' roles and clinical practice. It aims to help readers reflect on their own roles and responsibilities, considering boundaries within nursing generally and also within individual roles. It will examine hierarchies of professional practice, utilising current evidence and professional frameworks. There will also be a critical discussion of competencies for professional practice, clinical skills, advanced levels of practice and implications for training and objective assessments.

What is autonomy?

The term 'autonomy' is derived from the Greek language: *autos* (self) and *nomos* (rule or law). It originates when citizens made their own laws, thus suggesting that people are autonomous if they determine their own thoughts, decisions and actions, that is, if they 'rule' themselves. This can be contrasted with heteronomy, whereby a person is governed by someone else. Self-determination and the notion of freedom of choice seem common elements underpinning the concept of autonomy, although freedom of choice does not determine whether a person is autonomous, and other factors can influence autonomy.

Beauchamp and Childress (1994) propose that there are three essential factors in relation to autonomy:

- Liberty (freedom from controlling influences)
- Agency (the capacity for intentional action)
- Understanding (regarding disclosure of information)

A person whose autonomy is diminished is either under some control by others, or lacks the ability to reason about his own desires. In theory, it could be argued that in order for a person to be fully autonomous, there should be full understanding and freedom from distorting influences. However, in practice, this is unrealistic and it seems more appropriate to consider autonomy in terms of a sliding scale to determine the degree of autonomy a person may have.

The notion of rationality is pivotal to determining autonomy. If a person is autonomous they will desire and do what they judge to have good reason to do, therefore rationality facilitates the ability to choose and enables internal control of decisions.

In discussing autonomy, an important question to consider is whether it is the person or their actions that enable a person to be autonomous. This leads to consideration of an identity or a capacity account of autonomy, within which capacity is an account of an autonomous person and identity is an account of an autonomous action. Dworkin (1988) proposed that a capacity account of autonomy has greater validity since an identity account relates to specific acts over a short period of time, which can vary from one day to another, and therefore can potentially change determinations of autonomy. In contrast the capacity account of autonomy relates to a person's whole life, and not just isolated actions forming part of his life.

However, the capacity account does not appear to be sufficient, in that a person could have the capacity to formulate desires and make them effective, but is not necessarily autonomous throughout his life, even though his capacity remains constant. There are different influences or actions which could affect his autonomy, which places greater emphasis on the value of an identity account of autonomy.

Lindley (1986) proposes that it is impossible to be totally autonomous, and that it may be necessary to reach a certain level of autonomy. If this is valid, autonomy could be seen as a matter of degree. In the context of the nurse-patient relationships this is perhaps more appropriate, since other ethical principles have to be considered such as beneficence, nonmaleficence and paternalism.

Respect for autonomy may be regarded as acting in ways which do not undermine person's capacity for autonomy or ability to exercise autonomy. Autonomy may be impaired in some people with learning disabilities since they may lack the intellectual capacity to reason effectively, especially in new or complex situations. This is particularly important when considering a person's capacity to give informed consent for cancer treatment and/or clinical procedures.

Gillon (1986) argues that the only justifiable reason to override a person's autonomy is through paternalistic intervention acting in a person's best interests. However, such interventions should be carefully considered since impairment of a person's reasoning may be caused by other factors, such as information being distorted through misinterpretation, or poor communication skills when giving complex information.

Competence and autonomy

Lynch (1988) defines competence as having the capacity to make one's own decisions and the ability to understand the consequences of this. A core meaning of competence could be the ability to perform a task, the criteria of which would vary according to the task. In this way, the division between competence and incompetence would vary. Beauchamp and Childress (1994) suggest that competence should be viewed as a continuum concept, ranging from full competence through various levels of partial competence to full incompetence. However, in clinical practice health professionals may just try to determine whether a person is competent or incompetent.

The components of theoretical concepts of autonomy have been outlined, drawing comparisons between an identity and capacity account of autonomy, discussing which may be preferable and which has increased ethical validity. In applying this to clinical practice, it is useful to note the distinctions in order to determine whether it should be the person or their actions that determine autonomy. It also seems important to understand how a person's autonomy can be diminished by other factors, such as the use of coercion and manipulation, since this has particular relevance in clinical settings.

Determining mental capacity

It is estimated that as many as two million people in England may lack capacity to make certain decisions at a specific time (House of Lords 2014). Within this figure it is estimated that over one million people in England have learning disabilities and some will lack capacity to make certain decisions at times, up to 670,000 are living with dementia and may have issues of capacity, and many people will suffer from temporary mental impairment at some time (House of Lords 2014).

Defining mental capacity

The Mental Capacity Act (2005) was introduced as a legislative framework to determine the statutory rights of people who may lack capacity. It became fully effective in 2007 and applies to people aged sixteen years and over; however the Act only applies in England and Wales. Scotland has similar legislation, where issues of mental capacity are covered by the Adults with Incapacity (Scotland) Act 2000. In Northern Ireland capacity is covered by the Mental Health (Northern Ireland) Order 1986, although this is due to be updated by a new Mental Capacity Act (NMC 2015).

The vision was to empower people who may lack capacity by aiming to protect their rights, in particular emphasising their involvement in decision-making (House of Lords 2014). The Act is supported by the Mental Capacity Code of Practice (2015) which provides guidance and information, including recommendations for good practice.

The Mental Capacity Act 2005 states that

> A person lacks capacity in relation to a matter if at the material time he or she is unable to make a decision for himself or herself in relation to the matter because of an impairment of, or a disturbance in the functioning of, the brain or mind.
>
> (House of Lords 2014, 1)

This emphasises that capacity is time-specific, since a person may lack capacity to make a decision at one time but have the capacity to make the same decision at another time; in addition a person may be unable to make a decision about a specific matter, yet at the same time have the capacity to make a different decision about something else (House of Lords 2014). This is an important distinction and highlights the need to reassess capacity as appropriate.

The Mental Capacity Act (2005) is based on five principles:

1. *Presumption of capacity*: Capacity must be assumed unless it is established that they lack the capacity to make his or her own decisions.
2. *People have the right to be supported to make their own decisions*: People must be given all appropriate help before anyone can assume that they cannot make their own decisions.
3. *Making unwise decision should not be regarding as lack of capacity*: People should not be treated as unable to make a decision because they choose to make what is seen as an unwise decision.
4. *Act in the person's best interests*: Anything that is done for, or on behalf of, people without capacity must be done in the person's best interests.
5. *Ensure any action includes the least restrictions for people*: Anything that is done for, or on behalf of, people without capacity should be the least restrictive intervention in relation to the person's basic rights and freedom. (House of Lords 2014, NMC 2015)

The Mental Capacity Act provided legislative guidance for health professionals in relation to assessing mental capacity. In clinical practice this was particularly beneficial when informed consent was required and potential issues of mental capacity were highlighted. The introduction of local guidelines facilitated operational processes in clinical practice, providing clinicians with a clear direction of what actions to take, including who patients should be referred to for further assessment.

However, a House of Lords select committee (2014) stated that the Mental Capacity Act had not met expectations regarding its impact on individuals, suggesting that this was due to lack of awareness and understanding of the Act. It is important for nurses to be aware of the Mental Capacity Act and its implications, particularly if they are involved with obtaining informed consent. The NMC (2015, 6) emphasised that nurses must 'make sure that the rights and best interests of those who lack capacity are still at the centre of the decision-making process.'

Autonomy and the role of the nurse

The concept of autonomous nursing practice began with Florence Nightingale, who considered it essential to distinguish professional nursing practice from care provided by a layperson (Chitty 2007). Nowadays autonomy is considered synonymous with independence in nursing practice and a key factor in advanced nursing practice. However autonomy is generally poorly defined and understood (Gagnon et al. 2010). In healthcare there are different types of autonomy, including personal, clinical, organisational and professional autonomy, and although they may have similar features they have different contextual meanings (Gagnon et al. 2010). This seems an important factor to consider when trying to understand and interpret autonomy and nurses' roles.

The RCN (2010, 4) identifies an advanced nurse practitioner as someone who 'makes professionally autonomous decisions, for which he or she is accountable', which suggests that it is the nurses' actions regarding decision-making that are important rather than personal autonomy of the nurse. In contrast the NMC focus on nurses' accountability within professional practice and fail to mention professional autonomy (NMC 2008); although Keenan (1999) suggests that accountability may be regarded as a consequence of autonomy. Within nursing the meaning of accountability should be clear to all registered nurses, since it is set out in the professional code of conduct and relates to nurses' actions or omissions (NMC 2008); however interpreting the concept of autonomy is more complex.

As previously outlined, an important question to consider is whether it is the person or their actions that enable a person to be autonomous, leading to consideration of an identity (autonomous action) or a capacity (autonomous person) account of autonomy (Dworkin 1988). In applying this to clinical practice this may raise questions regarding possible distinctions between personal and professional autonomy, and the implications for professional practice.

The core characteristic of professional autonomy is freedom within the scope of practice to make independent decisions about nursing and patient care, which includes freedom in decision-making, independence and accountability (Gagnon et al. 2010). Although autonomy seems embodied within nurses' scope of practice, the nature of their work and relationships with patients and colleagues (Gagnon et al. 2010), the actualization of autonomy is multidimensional and complex given nurses' unique clinical roles and scope of clinical practice. Kramer et al. (2006) suggest three dimensions of professional autonomy:

1. Clinical/practice autonomy: independent, interdependent and accountable decision-making to benefit patients
2. Control over nursing practice autonomy: policy development by nurses to determine and direct nursing practice
3. Job/work autonomy: group decision-making at unit level to organise daily responsibilities and prioritise tasks

Batey and Lewis (1982) interpret autonomy as 'freedom to act' and propose that accountability cannot be considered in isolation from concepts of autonomy, responsibility and authority. Whilst all these factors seem relevant to professional accountability and autonomy, they seem to imply a theoretical hierarchy with different levels of accountability, autonomy and responsibilities as nurses progress from registration to advanced practice. If we consider that professional autonomy is synonymous with accountability, one could argue that greater professional autonomy results in a higher level of accountability, clinical responsibilities and clinical decision-making. However this must be underpinned by standards, competencies and corresponding levels of clinical responsibilities to ensure that the expansion of clinical practice to an advanced level is carefully regulated.

Lewis (2006) argues that nurses' training, clinical knowledge and understanding enable autonomous decision-making within the scope of professional practice; however, if approval or permission is required from someone more senior, this implies that the nurse is not acting with complete autonomy. In a systematic review of specialist and advanced practice roles, Lloyd-Jones (2005) stated that autonomy was one of the factors that facilitated role development and effective practice. This seems particularly true in oncology, where nurses associate greater knowledge and skills with increased autonomy and clinical responsibilities (Gagnon et al. 2010). This seems to reinforce considerations of a sliding scale of autonomy, together with accountability and responsibilities that could reflect the four levels of clinical practice from novice to expert.

It is also important to remember that nurses work as part of a multidisciplinary team; therefore collaboration with other professionals is in the best interests of the patient. Rafferty et al. (2001) found a strong synergistic association between teamwork and autonomy, identifying that nurses who displayed greater teamwork also had higher levels of autonomy and were more involved in decision-making.

Professional accountability and autonomy

As previously discussed, the NMC (2008) and previous professional regulatory bodies (UKCC 1992) focus on the accountability of nurses within clinical practice. However, Batey and Lewis (1982) propose that accountability cannot be considered in isolation from the concepts of autonomy (freedom to act), responsibility (a charge for which a person is answerable) and authority (the rightful power to act on the change). To address this, Walsh (1997) recommends that a clear distinction should be drawn between accountability (explaining and justifying actions based on sound clinical knowledge and transparent, logical and replicable decision-making) and responsibility (performance of tasks in an accurate and timely way through delegation). This suggests that accountability requires independent thought, therefore should be considered on a higher plane to responsibility. However the NMC Code of Practice (2008) links accountability and responsibility, stating that nurses are personally responsible for their own practice, answerable for their own acts and omissions regardless of advice or directions from another professional. This includes accountability for delegation of duties to another professional.

Autonomy and advanced nursing practice

The RCN (2010) definition of an advanced nurse practitioner includes the ability to make professionally autonomous decisions for which he or she is accountable.

Savage et al. (2004, 5) reported that whilst nurses' roles were expanding and responsibilities increasing, they were often 'bounded by the use of protocols', unlike other clinical colleagues. Although this study focused on the accountability of practice nurses, it has resonance with oncology specialist nurses, where nurses in a variety of different settings create protocols as guidance for their extended clinical practice, including nurse-led clinics (Farrell 2014).

Crossing boundaries in clinical practice

Crossing boundaries by taking on medical responsibilities is often difficult for nurses, even with the support of medical colleagues and managers. Barton et al. (2012) describe specialist nurses as the first product of the evolution of nursing, where the foundations of advanced nursing practice were set in the US. However the introduction of nurse practitioners was more controversial and challenging since it affected the relationship of nursing to other professions (Barton et al. 2012).

There is some evidence in the literature highlighting how nurses' roles are changing and the impact this may have on others. An ethnographic study of advanced nurse practitioners highlights their role in teaching junior medical and nursing staff, which is seen to promote advanced nurse practitioners as role models for both professions (Williamson et al. 2012). However, also shows how the role of advanced nurse practitioners may de-skill ward nurses by reducing their use of analytical skills, particularly when time is limited (Williamson et al. 2012).

Managers may also face difficulties when nurses expand their existing role if nurses' scope of practice and job description is not well defined (Torn and McNichol 1998); therefore clear lines of communication seem vital. Furthermore, since the majority of new cancer nursing roles have developed with little evidence of evaluation, it seems difficult to appreciate their impact and effectiveness on patients and cancer service delivery, and this may lead hospital managers to question their value.

Support for role development and advanced practice

From the literature, a systematic review identified different factors with influenced nurses' clinical roles; Jokiniemi et al. (2012) report that the organisational challenges rose from the newness of advanced roles, a lack of clarity with individual clinical roles, challenges within healthcare systems, and limited support and recognition from management, which had an adverse effect on the implementation of advanced practice roles. The authors found that a lack of support, together with high expectations and difficult working relationships within the multidisciplinary team, can potentially undermine the achievements of advanced nurse practitioners (Jokiniemi et al. 2012). Furthermore, without appropriate professional nursing support structures, advanced practitioners may seek their main professional mentorship from medical staff (Walters 1996).

A survey of eighty nurse practitioners reported the top three factors to help their role were linked to support from medical and nursing colleagues (Hupcey 1993).

This has been echoed by other studies where peer support was considered important for clinical nurse specialists (Hamric and Taylor, 1989) and support from physicians was required to develop clinical nurse specialist's roles (McFadden and Miller 1994). A study of 497 nurse practitioners illustrated that the presence and acceptance of support from professional colleagues facilitated their practice whilst the absence of support inhibited role development (Hayden et al. 1982). I found similar examples of this in my PhD research (Farrell 2014, 145), which the following quotes from nurse participants illustrate:

'I believe many people lack an understanding of the role and what it entails. Surprisingly the medical staff are the ones who recognise how much we do rather more than nursing colleagues' [clinical nurse specialist, CNS]

'My current role of CNS is reasonably valued but the change in role to [advanced nurse practitioner] ANP is not. There is no understanding of the role or its place . . .' [CNS]

There may also be issues in succession planning and career development:

'I struggle to get financial value and feel the pressure of the glass ceiling in terms of career development' [NC]

In my survey of 79 oncology specialist nurses in the UK who were running nurse-led clinics Farrell 2014), 48 nurses (60.8%) reported that they had a significant level of autonomy, whilst 12 (15.2%) reported their role was fully autonomous. However 16 (20.3%) had only 'some' autonomy and 2 (2.5%) relied on indirect supervision. There were mixed views on perceived level of autonomy about nurses' current role, with no comments by nurse practitioners and lead nurses. The following comment illustrates some of the conflict that can arise within organisations when developing new roles:

'We want our role to change from CNS to practitioner . . . [and] incorporate some elements of the practitioner role without eroding the core value of the CNS. Unfortunately organisations appear to be valuing the practitioner role at the expense of the CNS.' [CNS] (145)

Within the survey 56 (70.9%) nurses reported that barriers limited their practice. Three possible categories for barriers were outlined in the questionnaire: the organisation (n=31, 39.2%), the nursing directorate (n=13, 16.5%) and the medical directorate (n=18, 22.8%), plus an open category titled 'other barriers' (n=23, 29.1%) (see Figure 4.1). Included in other barriers were time, training, lack of support, the infrastructure/environment and lack of resources (Farrell et al. 2014). Specific barriers from managers were mainly in relation to the financial implications of role extension and development of new roles, which seems understandable in the current financial climate.

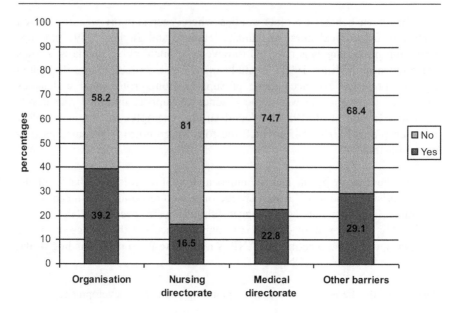

Figure 4.1 Barriers limiting nursing practice

However, nurses perceived that some medical colleagues placed obstructions in the way of their role development, which could hinder their clinical work. Some of this obstructive behaviour appeared to be due to a lack of understanding of changes in nurses' roles; however there were also reports of resistance by medical consultants to nurses developing their roles, which seems a more difficult obstacle to overcome:

> 'Due to this being a new role there are barriers at different levels with all disciplines although overall acceptance of the role has been good. I only work alongside the consultants that are accepting of ANP roles' [ANP] (148)
>
> 'One surgeon obstructive at times to developing staff / practice and very inconsistent in decision making generally so there are difficulties in agreeing vision for service at times' [NC]
>
> (Farrell et al. 2014, 148)

Doctor-nurse relationships have changed over time, with an increase in nurses' autonomy and involvement in clinical decision-making (Porter 1991, Stein et al. 1990). This goes some way to explain current tensions between the professions with the expansion of nurses' roles. Keddy et al. (1986) propose that this may threaten the medical profession since it represents a loss of power and status. Studies also suggest improvements over time with nurse-doctor relationships (Stein et al. 1990), particularly where junior doctors relied on senior nurses for advice, although some suggest that the 'doctor-nurse game' may still occur between nurses and medical consultants (Hughes 1988, Sweet and Norman 1995).

The importance of autonomy in advanced clinical practice

Autonomy and independence enabled nurses to use skills appropriate for their roles (Hupcey 1993), whilst nurses' self-confidence about their clinical ability, interpersonal skills and motivation facilitated role development (Hamric and Taylor 1989). Limitations in material and human resources were important barriers for nurses' roles (McFadden and Miller 1994; Sullivan et al. 1978), and also a lack of understanding of nurses' roles (Hamric and Taylor 1989).

It is widely considered that advanced practitioners are able to practice autonomously, with the freedom to make decisions about clinical practice, whilst accepting responsibility for their actions and being held to account for them (NHS 2007). Critical thinking is central to this process, allowing advanced practitioners to consider and analyse clinical evidence, including cases and situations, enabling a high level of clinical judgement and decision-making (NHS 2007). Mantzoukas et al. (2007) reports that this 'self-regulatory judgement' is key to practising autonomously since it demonstrates and ability to interpret, analyse, evaluate and draw inferences from this. In advanced practice there is often a high level of complex clinical decision-making, critical thinking and problem-solving, which sets it apart from other levels of clinical nursing practice, and this influences the ability to practice autonomously (NHS 2008).

Independence and autonomy in nurse-led clinics

Without research evidence it is difficult to know how independent nurse-led clinics are, and how autonomous nurses' practice is. Surveying 79 oncology specialist nurses who undertook nurse-led clinics revealed that 62 (79%) nurses reported that they could run their clinics independently from medical staff. However, doctors alone prescribed in 46 (58%) of nurse-led clinics, including all nurse-led clinics run by nurse practitioners and most of those run by CNSs (Farrell 2014) (see Figure 4.2). Although an increasing number of nurses independently prescribe medicines, an inability to prescribe within nurse-led clinics could limit the autonomy of nurses.

In addition, 49 (62%) nurses reported that they had 'cover' for their nurse-led clinic from another nurse (n=33, 42%), a doctor (n=12, 15%, or a pharmacist (n=3, 4%), which is shown in Table 4.1.

However some nurses reported a preference to run nurse-led clinics parallel to medical clinics, which provided nurses with the security of medical colleagues close by if needed, whilst others considered that joint clinics with medical consultants were the most appropriate for their clinical practice.

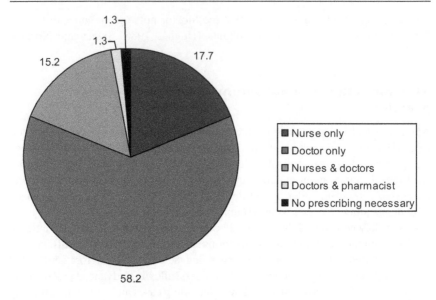

Figure 4.2 Prescribing within nurse-led clinics

Table 4.1 Autonomy within nurse-led clinics

	Independent		Also see doctors		Nurse prescribes		Doctor only prescribes		Cover available	
	n=	%	n=	%	n=	%	n=	%	n=	%
CNS	33	76.7	19	44.2	5	11.6	30	69.8	25	58.1
NP	5	71.4	1	14.3	0	0	6	85.7	5	71.4
ANP	4	80	2	40	2	40	0	0	4	80
NC	8	88.9	6	66.7	3	33.3	3	33.3	4	44.4
LN	6	75	1	12.5	3	37.5	3	37.5	6	75
CN	5	83.3	2	33.3	1	16.7	3	50	5	83.3

An ethnographic observational study of nurse-led chemotherapy clinics showed disparities in nurses' autonomy across four geographical areas in England (Farrell et al. 2014). In some locations nurses do not have written protocols and adopt similar clinical responsibilities and autonomy to medical staff in relation to prescribing and clinical management of patients. In contrast, other locations work to strict protocols which guide their scope of practice within their clinics. In some cases protocols for nurse-led clinics were written by medical consultants, which placed severe restrictions on their clinical practice and independent prescribing within nurse-led clinics (Farrell et al. 2014). In addition some nurses restrict their own autonomy by the way they work within the nurse-led clinics. Examples of this included the way nurses structured their consultations with patients, or their own lack of self-confidence with aspects of their extended role such as clinical examination skills and independent prescribing.

Uncertainties about autonomy and advanced practice

Some nurses seem to associate increased autonomy with independent clinical decision-making and taking on medical responsibilities, perceiving that the medicalization of nursing roles equates to advanced nursing practice (Farrell et al. 2014). In contrast some nurses recognised that this should be combined with nursing, rather than doctor-nurse substitution. However some nurses regard advanced nursing practice as a 'skill set', associated more with certain courses and qualifications than responsibilities within nurses' roles. Observing nurses in nurse-led chemotherapy clinics, it seems that the way nurses use their personal autonomy directly influences autonomy of their role, and one of the greatest influences appears to be nurses' confidence, although nurses' perceptions are underpinned by their personal beliefs (Farrell 2014).

Summary

Although the NMC (2008) focuses on accountability within the code of conduct and regulations for professional practice, responsibilities, competencies and autonomy are closely inter-linked. The concept of autonomy is not straightforward and there are many layers embedded within it, which have ethical, practical, personal and professional implications for nurses and other health professionals. Nurses must also have a working knowledge of the Mental Capacity Act (2005) and its implications regarding mental capacity.

Crossing boundaries by taking on medical responsibilities is often difficult for nurses, even with support of medical colleagues and managers. Barton et al. (2012) describe specialist nurses as the first product of the evolution of nursing, where the foundations of advanced nursing practice were set in the US. However the introduction of nurse practitioners was more controversial and challenging since it affected the relationship of nursing to other professions (Barton et al. 2012). There were subtle examples of this within my survey (Farrell 2014), which suggest that when nurses expand their clinical roles some doctors may feel that nurses are 'treading on their toes'; in addition, other nurses may feel threatened when the roles of their colleagues change.

References

Adults with Incapacity (Scotland) Act. (2000). Available at: www.legislation.gov.uk/asp/2000/4/contents [last accessed 16.02.2015].

Barton TD, Bevan L, Mooney G. (2012). Advanced nursing 1: The development of advanced nursing roles. *Nursing Times.* 108(24): 18–20.

Batey M, Lewis F. (1982). Clarifying autonomy and accountability. Part 1 *Journal of Nursing Administration*. September: 13–18.

Beauchamp TL, Childress JF. (1994). *Principles of Biomedical Ethics*, 4th.ed. Oxford, Oxford University Press.

Chitty K. (2007). Educational patterns in nursing. In *Professional nursing. Concepts and challenges*, 5th ed (KK Chitty and BP Black, eds.). St Louis, Saunders Elseiver. 161–187.

Dworkin G. (1988). *The Theory and Practice of Autonomy*. Cambridge, Cambridge University Press.

Farrell C. (2014). *An exploration of oncology nurse specialists' roles in nurse-led chemotherapy clinics*. Unpublished PhD thesis, University of Manchester.

Gagnon L, Bakker D, Montgomery P, Palkovits JA. (2010). Nurse autonomy in cancer care. *Cancer Nursing*. 33(3): 21–28.

Gillon R. (1986). Do doctors owe a special duty of beneficence to their patients? *Journal of Medical Ethics*. 12: 171–173.

Hamric AB, Taylor JW. (1989). Role development of the CNS. In *The clinical nurse specialist in theory and practice*, 2nd ed (Hamric and Spross, eds.). Philadelphia, WB Saunders.

Hayden ML, Davies LR, Clore ER. (1982). Facilitators and Inhibitors of the emergency nurse practitioner role. *Nursing Research*. 31: 294–299.

House of Lords Select Committee. (2014). *Valuing every voice, respecting every right: Making the case for the Mental Capacity Act: The government's response to the House of Lords Select Committee Report on the Mental Capacity Act 2005*. London, HMSO.

Hughes D. (1988). When nurse knows best: some aspects of the nurse/doctor interaction in a casualty department, *Sociology of Health and Illness*. 10(1): 1–22.

Hupcey JE. (1993). Factors and work settings that may influence nurse practitioner practice. *Nursing Outlook*. 41: 181–185.

Jokiniemi K, Pietilä AM, Kylmä J, Haatainen K. (2012). Advanced nursing roles: a systematic review. *Nursing Health Science*. 14(3): 421–31. doi: 10.1111/j.1442–2018.2012.0 0704.x.

Keenan J. (1999). A concept analysis of autonomy. *Journal of Advanced Nursing*. 29(3): 556–562.

Kramer M, Maguire P, Schamlenberg C. (2006). Excellence through evidence: the what, when, and where of clinical autonomy. *Journal of Nursing Adm*. 36(10): 479–491.

Keddy B, Jones-Gillis M, Jacobs P, Burton H, Rogers, M. (1986). The doctor-nurse relationship: an historical perspective. *Journal of Advanced Nursing*. 11: 745–753.

Lewis FM. (2006). Autonomy in nursing. *Ishikawa Journal of Nursing*. 3(2): 1–6.

Lindley R. (1986). *Autonomy*. London, Macmillan.

Lloyd-Jones M. (2005). Role development and effective practice in specialist and advanced practice roles in acute hospital settings: systematic review and meta-synthesis. *Journal of Advanced Nursing*. 49(2): 191–209.

Lynch MT. (1988). The nurse's role in the biotherapy of cancer: clinical trials and informed consent. *Oncology Nursing Forum*. Supplement to 15(6): 23–27.

Mantzoukas S, Watkinson S. (2007). Review of advanced nursing practice: the international literature and developing the generic features. *Journal of Clinical Nursing*. 16: 28–37.

McFadden EA, Miller MA. (1994). Clinical nurse specialists practice: facilitators and barriers. *Clinical Nurse Specialist*. 8: 27–33.

Mental Capacity Act. (2005). Available at: www.legislation.gov.uk/ukpga/2005/9/contents [last accessed 16.02.2015].

Mental Capacity Act Code of Practice. (2015). Available at: www.justice.gov.uk/downloads/protecting-the-vulnerable/mca-code-practice-0509.pdf [last accessed 16.02.2015].

The Mental Health (Northern Ireleand) Order. (1986). Number 595. Available at: http://www.legislation.gov.uk/nisi/1986/595/pdfs/uksi_19860595_en.pdf [last accessed 23.05.2015].

Nursing and Midwifery Council. (2008). *The Code: Standards of conduct, performance and ethics for nurses and midwives.* London. NMC.

Nursing and Midwifery Council. (2015). *The Code: Professional standards of practice and behavior for nurses and midwives.* London, NMC.

NHS Education for Scotland. (2007). *Working with individuals with cancer, their families and carers. Professional development framework for nurses and allied health professionals. Core level.* Edinburgh, NHS.

NHS Education for Scotland. (2008). *Working with individuals with cancer, their families and carers: Professional development framework for nurses, specialist and advanced levels.* Edinburgh, NHS.

NMC. (2015). *Consent.* Available at: http://www.nmc-uk.org/Nurses-and-midwives/Regulation-in-practice/Regulation-in-Practice-Topics/consent/ [last accessed 16.02.2015].

Porter, S. (1991). A participant observation study of power relations between nurses and doctors in a general hospital. *Journal of Advanced Nursing.* 16: 728–735.

Rafferty AM, Ball J, Aiken LH. (2001). Are teamwork and professional autonomy compatible, and do they result in improved hospital care? *Quality in Health Care.* 10 (Supplement II): 32–37.

RCN. (2010). *RCN Competencies: Advanced nurse practitioners.* London. RCN.

Savage J, Moore L. (2004). RCN Research reports: Interpreting accountability. *An ethnographic study of practice nurses, accountability and multidisciplinary team decision-making in the context of clinical governance.* London. RCN.

Stein L, Watts DT, Howell T. (1990). The doctor-nurse game revisited. *New England Journal of Medicine.* 322(8): 546–549.

Sullivan JA, Dachelet CZ, Sultz HA, Henry M, Carrol HD. (1978). Overcoming barriers to employment and utilization of the nurse practitioner. *American Journal of Public Health.* 68: 1097–1103.

Sweet SJ, Norman IJ. (1995). The nurse-doctor relationship: a selective literature review. *Journal of Advanced Nursing.* 22: 165–170.

Torn A, McNichol E. (1998). A qualitative study utilizing focus group to explore the role and concept of the nurse practitioner. *Journal of Advanced Nursing.* 27: 1202–1211.

United Kingdom Central Council for Nursing. (1992). *Code of Professional Practice.* London, UKCC.

Walsh, M. (1997). Accountability and intuition: justifying nursing practice. *Nursing Standard.* 11 (23): 39–41.

Walters AJ. (1996). Being a clinical nurse consultant: a hermeneutic phenomenological reflection. *Int. Journal of Nursing Practice.* 2: 2–10.

Williamson S, Twelvetree T, Thompson J, Beaver K. (2012). An ethnographic study exploring the role of ward-based advanced nurse practitioners in an acute medical setting. *Journal of Advanced Nursing.* 68(7): 1579–1588.

Chapter 5

Non-medical prescribing

Elaine Lennan

History of non-medical prescribing

The introduction of non-medical prescribing (NMP), that is, the prescribing of medicines by health-care professionals other than doctors, was first discussed in the United Kingdom (UK) in 1986 (DHSS 1986). Almost thirty years later it is now an exciting opportunity for nurses and others, made possible by government policy and supported by the Nursing and Midwifery Council (NMC) (Department of Health [DOH] 2000a, DOH 2003a). The main aim of the renewed policy was to streamline access to medicines for patients and best utilise skills and knowledge of all health professionals, recognising in modern health care a doctor may not be the most appropriate person to supply a medicine or product (DOH 2003a). However the initial reviews were only a beginning. In addition to these early changes further amendments to legislation have recently taken place which extend this scope further, as seen in Table 5.1.

Implementation of NMP

From the early enthusiasm of the beginning of the 21st century it has actually taken much longer than anticipated to develop non-medical prescribing. An initial target of 10,000 nurses able to prescribe by 2004 fell well short of the actual 2,000 nurses registered to prescribe at that time (DOH 2003a). However the last five years have seen a general acceptance of NMP and in 2011 figures suggest there were over 18,000 nurses registered to prescribe (Latter and Blenkinsopp 2011). Recent numbers obtained from the NMC in December 2014 are detailed in Table 5.2, indicating over 32,000 independent nurse prescribers.

However, the slow progression for training and implementation was troublesome on three counts:

1. The ambitious targets lacked strategic planning for implementation.
2. The rapid changes in legislation unnerved many in all professions.
3. The far-reaching scope of the NMP initiative exceeded anywhere else in the world, causing some unrest within the medical profession.

(Lennan 2014)

Table 5.1 Timeline of recent changes to prescribing legislation

Date	Milestone	Source
1999	Review of supply and administration of medicines	DOH (1999b) Review of supply and administration of medicines, Final report. HMSO, London.
2000	First widespread consultation on proposals to widen scope of prescribing	DOH (2000b) Consultation on proposals to extend nurse prescribing. HMSO, London
May 2001	First announcement about extension of nurse prescribing to cover a range of conditions	DOH publications and statistics online (2001). Patients to get quicker access to medicines [Online] 24 October 2006, http://www.doh.gov.uk
Feb 2002	Training for first cohort of independent nurse prescribers begins Scope: Extended but still limited formulary known as Nurse Prescribers Extended Formulary (NPEF)	DOH publications and statistics online (2002). More prescribing power to nurses [Online] 24 October 2006, http://www.doh.gov.uk
April 2002	Training of first cohorts complete and those qualified now able to prescribe from NPEF	www.nmc.org.uk [Online] 24 October 2006
April 2003	Supplementary prescribing for nurses/pharmacists introduced. Plans for other allied health professionals to train as supplementary prescribers, e.g. physio, optometrists, podiatrists Scope: All licensed medicines within a clinical management plan	DOH (2003b) Supplementary prescribing by nurses and pharmacists within the NHS in England. HMSO, London
May 2006	Further extension of scope. Independent nurse prescribers are able to prescribe any licensed medicines (including some controlled drugs) within their own level of competence. Pharmacist independent prescribers able to prescribe any licensed medicine with the exception of controlled drugs within their level of competence	DOH (2006) Improving access to medicines: A guide to implementing nurse and pharmacist independent prescribing within the NHS in England. HMSO, London
April 2012	Removes the restrictions applied to controlled drugs (excluding cocaine, diamorphine or dipipanone for the treatment of addiction)	Home Office circular 009/2012

Table 5.2 Number of nurse prescribers to date (NMC 2014)

Effective practitioners by qualification	Number
V100] – Community Practitioner Nurse Prescriber	35,586
V150] – Community Practitioner Nurse Prescriber	2,190
V200] – Nurse Independent Prescriber	1,366
V300] – Nurse Independent / Supplementary Prescriber	31,115

In addition during these changes, the Harold Shipman enquiry was unnerving to the medical professional, as noted in the quote below;

> I think given the extreme, well I think its extreme, response, regulatory response, we have seen to the isolated insanity of Shipman it is, bizarre to permit a huge body of people who have been subject to substantially less pharmacologic training, the authority to prescribe those drugs.
>
> (Lennan 2014 p 417)

Indeed the British Medical Association in 2005 reacted in horror and voted solidly for the 'slowest possible progress' (Hawkes 2005). Despite these barriers NMP has been introduced and is now well established within health care.

Literature review of NMP

There is still not a vast amount of literature in relation to the effectiveness and impact of NMP. Studies that exist examine different setting and different scopes of prescribing, making comparisons difficult, and formularies at the time of many of the studies were too restrictive for some to have the impact the government required in radically transforming the health service. Recent legislative reform has since widened the formulary.

The nurses' view

The NMP movement is young, and consequently the most researched area of non-medical prescribing is the nurses' experience and viewpoint. There is emerging evidence to support the benefit of non-medical prescribing practice in a variety of clinical settings, but the evidence is minimal. Most of the research to date has been based in primary care, and it is clear the evidence depicts an overall positive experience regarding non-medical prescribing. These benefits include time saving, increased satisfaction, increased status and autonomy and increased self-esteem (Luker et al. 1997, Basford 2003, Lewis-Evans and Jester 2004, Bradley et al. 2005, Baird 2001, Hall et al. 2006, Latter et al. 2005, Clegg 2006, Scrafton et al. 2012, Pearce and Winter 2014).

A paper by Latter et al. (2005) endorses much of the above. This paper, a government-funded evaluation of extended formulary independent nurse prescribing, describes a strong viewpoint that prescribing has had a positive impact on the quality of the care given, by improving access to medicines and by making better use of the nurses' skills. It further supports the notion of increased autonomy and greater satisfaction, an effect reinforced by Courtenay and Carey (2007) and Courtenay et al. (2007). These additional large national evaluations found nurses prescribing in practice confidently and independently with the majority (84%) based in primary care. Similarly and without exception a survey by Green and Courtenay (2008) reported only positive experiences of non-medical prescribing in mental health practice. This small survey of 10 practitioners agreed with the benefits already stated but added the potential to unlock nurse-led services and influence the multi-professional team.

However some studies have indicated barriers do exist and need to be addressed, in particular breaking down organisational restraints and developing ongoing supportive strategies to facilitate further developments of NMP. These barriers featured in the first studies and continue in the more recent reports (Luker et al. 1997, Basford 2003, Lewis-Evans and Jester 2004, Bradley et al. 2005, Baird 2001, Hall et al. 2006, Latter et al. 2005, Clegg 2006, Scrafton et al. 2012, Courtenay and Carey 2007, Courtenay et al. 2007, Green and Courtenay 2008).

Lewis-Evans and Jester (2004) highlight a pressure to prescribe and issues regarding accountability. Pressure to prescribe came from all angles. The participants described the patients' desire to have what they wanted, not what they needed; the managers expected the nurses to take on that role; and the pharmaceutical industry pushed their products constantly. Despite this all, the participants felt they worked from a basis of evidence-based practice and were able to resist the pressure. Scrafton et al. (2012) clearly felt the skill was a senior nursing role, and resisting pressure would suggest this. Pearce and Winter (2013) most recently have audited prescribing practice amongst community workers and found good prescribing practices but still noted a concern about a lack of support from the organisation and continuing professional development.

The doctors' view

Initially in response to the proposals to extend non-medical prescribing the British Medical Association reacted with dismay and asked for urgent dialogue with the Department of Health (Hawkes 2005, Buckley et al. 2006, Day 2005, Salvage 2006). Though much commentary is available expressing concerns about non-medical prescribing, only a few studies address the medical viewpoint.

The earliest study by Luker et al. (1997) examined GPs' views of the nurse prescriber's formulary and found concerns about the constraints of the formulary. Indeed some expressed disappointment at the limitations and supported an extension of the list to include antibiotics and drugs to manage chronic illness. Interestingly in this early development of non-medical prescribing before an open formulary had even been suggested, two of the doctors felt that nurses, like doctors, should be accountable and limitations on practice should be based on knowledge and competence and not the external control of a formulary. Hay and Bradley (2004) explored the attitudes of the multidisciplinary team with regard to supplementary prescribing and found confusion and a lack of awareness of supplementary prescribing by the doctors. Once concept of supplementary prescribing was explained, many thought it was legitimizing what was already happening in practice, and many others thought with training there was no reason that nurses should not take on a prescribing role. Others questioned a need if a doctor was available and could see a 'filling a gap' role but emphasised the importance of good communication and team working. Buckley et al. (2006) found similar views amongst doctors. Interviews revealed that the concept of non-medical prescribing would save time and hassle. The need to follow guidelines was reiterated as was working as a team, but as with Hay and Bradley (2004), doctors in this study felt it was formalising current practice.

Avery et al. (2007) evaluated non-medical prescribing in a regional health authority and found the doctor-nurse relationship to be particularly important. Where a relationship was well established, non-medical prescribing flourished to its full potential, however when lacking, nurses were restricted in their practice. Avery et al. (2007) suggest that the evidence for this is in the GP practice, where close proximity working prevailed, and point to the lack of development in the acute hospitals, where many different professionals interacted. Latter et al. (2005) concurs with this. Interviewed GPs were very positive about the advent of nurse prescribing but linked their views to the nurses they worked with and knew rather than a general endorsement of nurse prescribing. In contrast to Buckley's (2006) findings of time saved and less hassle, GPs in the Latter et al. (2005) study found nurses were slower in their consultations and more protocol-driven. In addition concerns were expressed by GPs about their own potential role erosion, though this was acknowledged to be diminishing as they understood nurse prescribing better. Courtenay and Berry (2007) compared the views of doctors and nurses in an attempt to understand each other's concerns. Interestingly both groups identified more advantages than disadvantages. In contrast to the Avery et al. (2007) study, none of the doctors here valued improved doctor-nurse relationships in terms of non-medical prescribing, whereas 25 per cent of nurses thought it to be an advantage. Both nurses and doctors agreed that non-medical prescribing improved nurses' ability to meet patients' needs in terms of information-giving, approachability and accessibility.

Despite the initial reaction of the BMA, some individual doctors supported the further development of non-medical prescribing. Earwicker (2005), a GP with experience of nurse prescribing, declared it safe and that its introduction had been helped by strong and open clinical teams supporting nurses throughout their training and beyond. This stance is echoed by Richmond (2005), who argues that an experienced and qualified nurse is better placed to take on extended roles such as prescribing than a house officer with little experience, and supports the notion of close team working. More recently Courtenay (2008) has reported that despite strengthening educational standards, the medical profession still has concerns and misunderstandings about the role. She declares that to maximise the benefits of non-medical prescribing, nurses need to feel supported in practice, and there is a need for a continued education and information feedback to the medical profession. Most recently Stenner et al. (2012) found GPs supportive of the prescribing nurses with whom they worked. However, the acceptance of nurse prescribing in general was conditional upon the selection of nurses with appropriate experience and training. Not all nurses were considered to meet these requirements or, as non-prescribing nurse participants demonstrated, were ready to undertake this role.

The patients' view

Patients are important stakeholders in any service. Luker et al. (1998) interviewed a sample of 148 patients who had been involved with a nurse prescriber. A positive experience was relayed by the majority of the respondents, and some held the view that the nurse was best placed to deliver that aspect of their care, either because they knew the patient very well or knew the required drug/product in depth. Other positive evaluations included the ongoing development and longevity of the nurse-patient relationship, and the nurse's style and approachability. This sometimes led to discussions around health issues that they might not have otherwise raised.

Similarly Brooks et al. (2001a) explored patients' perceptions of nurse prescribing. Here several nurse prescribers were asked to identify five patients for whom they had prescribed. Fifty patients were recruited and interviewed, either in person or over the telephone. Whilst there is an obvious prejudice, given the nurses recruited their own patients, the respondents gave similar accounts to the Luker et al. (1998) study. Benefits cited of nurse prescribing include effective use of time, timeliness, convenience and continuity (Brooks et al. 2001b). Both studies were based in primary care, but the cohorts were different. Luker et al. (1998) describe their sample as high users of nursing services, whereas the sample of Brooks et al. (2001a) were low users. The findings from these studies complement each other, and it appears that the frequency of exposure to a nurse prescriber did not affect the viewpoint of the users.

Latter et al. (2005) similarly found that patients were generally positive in their experience of nurse prescribing. Patients were surveyed by questionnaire following an observed consultation in a variety of clinical settings. Particular weight was given to the quicker access to the medicine when prescribed by a nurse, though when specifically asked, no preference was indicated by the majority between seeing a doctor or a nurse. However several did state they would prefer to see a doctor about certain conditions, indicating the importance of choice. This supports the findings of Brooks et al. (2001b). No information is given as to whether the different clinical settings found different levels of satisfaction or whether the 'certain' conditions requiring a doctor were common to particular settings. Having said that, the patients indicated confidence in the nurse's ability to prescribe and were generally satisfied with having their information needs met. Interestingly the observed consultations as part of this research highlighted the possibility that though nurses are consistently giving information about some aspects of medicines they are prescribing, they may be less consistent at information-giving about other aspects, such as risks versus benefits and side effects. This perhaps highlights a mismatch regarding patient satisfaction, in that they are satisfied with what they were told but do not know what they should have been told and therefore cannot be dissatisfied!

A different approach to the patient view on nurse prescribing was noted in a study by Berry et al. (2006). The aim of this study was to assess the views of those not yet exposed to a nurse prescriber. A convenience sample of 74 members of the public was recruited from a London railway station. The individuals were asked to complete a five-page validated questionnaire divided into four categories; attitudes, information needs, confidence in doctor or nurse and experience to date. Whilst acknowledging potential limitations, such as the convenience sample of volunteers and the exploratory nature of the study, the indications were very positive towards nurse prescribing supporting the findings of Luker et al. (1998), Brooks et al. (2001a) and Latter et al. (2005). Respondents stated they would have confidence in the nurse prescribing the best medicine and stated that they would be very likely to take that medicine. No concerns were elicited regarding the nurse's status and the most important factor for the individual was a full explanation of the side effects. Most felt this was a remit of the nursing role. Similarly Gerard et al. (2014) conducted a large audit of patient preferences with regard to seeing a prescribing nurse or the GP. Patients favoured seeing their own GP for minor illnesses but valued the consultation style of the nurse. This offers some insight about how best to use the prescribing nurse in primary care and highlights the need to engage all stakeholders in medicines management.

Only one study has examined the patient view of pharmacist prescribing in secondary care. Fitzpatrick et al. (2008) interviewed 40 patients whilst inpatients. A distinct lack of awareness about the hospital pharmacist's role was noted, though the potential for the pharmacist to have a prescribing role was viewed positively. All thought the pharmacists had superior knowledge about medicines than other health professionals but some felt the need to have a doctor in the background and would be more reassured if a doctor referred them to a pharmacist for management of their condition.

Non-medical prescribing in the acute setting

The acute setting is yet to be studied in depth and warrants investment in research. This is important as there is a vast difference in the structure and culture of the acute setting versus the primary care setting. Organisational barriers such as collection of prescription pads, repeat prescriptions and lack of access to medical record documentation as seen in primary care are potentially irrelevant to acute care, but other barriers may emerge in the acute setting. Non-medical prescribers in the acute setting will be equally accountable for their practice, but one could argue there is more availability of immediate support from colleagues in hospital settings than in the community.

There are inherent differences in the illness profile of individuals at home compared with hospital. The acute setting is increasingly for specialist services and acutely unwell individuals, be it a new diagnosis or exacerbation of a chronic illness. These are fundamental differences that are likely to impact the implementation and evaluation of non-medical prescribing. This emphasises the need for research into the value of non-medical prescribing in acute settings. The studies by Buckley et al. (2006) and Fitzpatrick et al. (2008) have begun this process, but given the huge array of specialities available within acute trusts, other settings must also be investigated. Of particular note in the Buckley et al. (2006) study were the inter- and intra-professional tensions regarding established roles or the potential for extended roles. This is confirmed in a later study by Cooper et al. (2008). This clearly suggests that involvement of all stakeholders, be it those developing an enhanced role or those being disenfranchised, is necessary to determine and develop the strategic direction for NMP implementation.

Goswell and Siefers (2009) and Crew (2010) describe their own practice in acute ward settings and conclude that they currently prescribe more than their counterparts in medicine and offer enhanced patient care through safe and timely access to medicines, increased patient involvement in decisions and collaborative team working. They further stress that prescribing never occurs in isolation, but use the multidisciplinary team (MDT) for support. Jones (2009, 2011) recognising the lack of research in acute care developed an evaluative case study. Findings show an equivalence between doctors and prescribing nurses, and likewise Poonawala and Grahem-Clarke (2007) demonstrated enhanced practice without compromising safety in the ITU setting.

Finally Scrafton et al. (2012) examined prescribing in secondary care and found clear benefits, but again it is disappointing that organisational constraints continue to provide barriers. In addition this study found that prescribing nurses considered that the ability to prescribe was exclusively a remit of an experienced nurse and that nurses were unsupported by their managers. They offer explanations to this that many NMPs are managed by non-prescribers. This makes appraisal and development needs difficult to understand.

NMP and cancer

There is a very small amount of research related to cancer care. A large national survey of Macmillan nurses investigated their views in relation to nurse prescribing (Ryan-Woolley et al. 2007). The nurses surveyed were working in all settings, with 11 per cent being community prescribers and 10 per cent independent prescribers. Further examination revealed a distinct reluctance to prescribe in any setting, with reasons given as lack of mentorship, insufficient focus and depth of training and organisational constraints. In addition one quarter could not see any benefits to the patient by becoming a prescribing nurse.

A paper by Fitzsimmons et al. (2005) examined the chemotherapy setting in relation to nurse-led care. Whilst not explicitly examining prescribing, prescribing is implied, in order to deliver a nurse-led service for chemotherapy. This study explored the perspectives of people affected by cancer and health-care professionals about the current medically led service and proposed nurse-led chemotherapy. As this was discussing views on a potential service, a difficulty was noted in users conceptualizing what a nurse-led service would entail. Users had firm views on traditional medical and nursing roles and in reflecting on their care found great difficulty in conceptualizing how changing these roles might enhance their care. An example is given around nurse prescribing. It was explained to users that whilst the decision about what treatment regimen to give would always be made by the medical oncologist, the nurse would continue that treatment protocol and prescribe the actual treatment at each visit. As the patient experience was context-specific, it was thought to be difficult to envisage a redesign of the service. However views of patients were mixed. Some expressed they would be quite satisfied with nurse-led care, other patients felt reassured if the doctor was 'in the background', and others stated they would not be happy. No figures are given to inform these views, but this supports the findings of Fitzpatrick (2008) in that exposure to new practice was important in understanding the implications. Farrell (2014) has evaluated an advanced nurse practitioner-led clinic in breast cancer, which confirmed patients' acceptability of nurse-led clinics.

Fitzsimmons et al. (2005) also examines the health professionals' views by interviewing 22 health-care professionals who worked within the same cancer network, some confined to one Trust, others working across three Trusts. These professionals held mixed views about nurse-led chemotherapy. Medical staff believed it to be a useful development, whilst others, mainly nurses, felt there would be a loss of the nursing role. A major finding of this study was the use of the term 'doctor-nurse substitution.' This was noted across both the service users and health professionals. Participants envisaged that nurses would be working in relative isolation, making sole decisions about treatment plans, rather than working in separate but complementary roles. The authors recommend a mixed economy model where nurses work in an enhanced therapeutic role within the multidisciplinary team. This, interestingly, supports the findings of the national evaluation of prescribing by Latter et al. (2005) in that prescribing was considered to work well when it occurred within a team context. Others have similarly found team working beneficial (Humphries and Green, 2000, Otway 2002, Bradley and Nolan 2007, Hay and Bradley 2004).

However, Fitzsimmons et al. (2005) add a caution that the success of these new roles within the team will depend on all stakeholders feeling confident that the highest quality of care is being delivered. The Fitzsimmons et al. paper (2005) demonstrates a degree of contrast to the direction of health policy (DOH 2009) in that the nurses specifically did not want to take on prescribing roles. Some smaller site-specific reports have been reported. Bowden and Horne (2011) describe a joint clinic with the oncologist specifically focussing on tyrosine kinase inhibitors management, which showed an overall acceptance by patients. Likewise an audit by Holland et al. (2014) demonstrated clear adherence to legislative frameworks by a single practitioner in a lung cancer clinic reassuring colleagues of the acceptability of NMP.

Finally Lennan (2014) specifically studied NMP in a chemotherapy clinic and found it to be an acceptable model of care with some caveats. The need to develop good working relationships with the MDT was paramount, as was the need to avoid working in isolation. The study suggests local adaptations will be necessary to address local needs, but these two fundamental requirements should not be compromised.

Practice implications

Cancer services have been fortunate over the past decade to have clear DOH policy to guide services (DOH 2007, DOH 2009). This is much needed, given the huge rise in demand for cancer services due to increased incidence, early diagnosis, better outcomes of therapy, availability of further therapy, new drugs, new technologies and an aging population.

Within these policies, work to improve the throughput and efficiency of the clinics and the role of professionals within these processes has also been examined. The NHS Cancer Plan (DOH 2000c) clearly outlined new roles for various health professionals and urged a critical examination of the workforce. Similarly the Nursing Contribution to Cancer Care (DOH 2000a) and Making a Difference (DOH 1999a) set out new roles for nurses (and allied health professionals) and amongst other things support the initiative of ordering tests and holding caseloads. Maturing this thinking, the Cancer Reform Strategy (DOH 2007) strengthened the commitment to new roles and new ways of working; however policy directives may not always easily translate into practice developments.

There is no doubt that services have struggled with provision in that cancer clinics and chemotherapy services remain overstretched, with long waiting times and inefficient services (Oliver 2002). Policy documents addressed this challenge by clearly outlining new roles for various health professionals, however, in general cancer services, an emphasis has been placed on patient-triggered follow-up and nurse-led follow-up clinics (DOH 2013). Clearly being a non-medical prescriber can enhance this, for example prescribing bowel preparations and anaemia remedies in colorectal cancer or hormones in breast cancer.

In chemotherapy services the lack of prescriptive authority for non-doctors has clearly hampered progress. The National Chemotherapy Advisory Group (NCAG) report fully endorses the development of nurse-led chemotherapy clinics, and this is a considered and welcome acknowledgment of the chemotherapy nursing workforce (DOH 2009). However the inability to prescribe has always been a major source of frustration (Fitzsimmons et al. 2005, Lennan 2014). Indeed, some chemotherapy clinics exist where the nurse will assess the patient, make decisions about treatment, including alterations and additional drugs, but then wait for the doctor to prescribe (Farrell 2014). This is little more than a prescription-writing exercise, as the nurse has made all the decisions. This practice arguably confuses accountability and potentially hides the contribution of the nurse. The prescriptive authority now granted to the nursing profession allows nurses to clearly illuminate a contribution, and this is supported by the UK Oncology Nursing Society (UKONS) position statement for nurse-led chemotherapy, which regards prescriptive authority as the gold standard. In addition, this skill, on implementation, paves the way for the development of robust services on which to develop further research in cancer services on a mass scale.

Current legislation

Given the recent rapidly changing legislation, it is important to understand the current position with regard to NMP. The current legislation allows two forms of non-medical prescribing, known as independent nurse prescribing and supplementary prescribing, however there are other ways to supply medicines to patients, and practitioners should consider carefully what best suits their needs. Table 5.3 outlines the differences.

Table 5.3 The legal mechanisms for supplying medicines

Legal mechanism	Description
Patient-specific direction	The traditional written instruction from a doctor, dentist or other prescriber for medicines to be supplied or administered to a named patient.
Exemptions	Specific exemptions for particular professional groups from the provisions of medicines legislation which would normally prevent them from supplying or administering medicines. Some exemptions require an additional professional qualification.
Patient group directions	Written instruction for the supply and/or administration of a licensed medicine (or medicines) in an identified clinical situation, where the patient may or may not be individually identified before presenting for treatment. PGDs can only be used by specified registered health-care professionals.
Supplementary prescribing	Voluntary prescribing partnership between the independent prescriber (doctor or dentist) and supplementary prescriber, to implement an agreed patient-specific clinical management plan (CMP), with the patient's agreement.
Independent prescribing	Allows trained nurses and pharmacist prescribers to prescribe any medicine for any medical condition that they are competent to treat. Optometrist prescribers can prescribe any licensed medicine for conditions connected with the eye that they are competent to treat.

National Prescribing Centre (NPC) 2012

An example from practice is the management of emergency sepsis. It may well be more appropriate and cost effective to develop a list of named nurses competent in the use of a patient group direction for an antibiotic to manage neutropenic sepsis and achieve a one-hour door-to-needle time, than to put every nurse through a non-medical prescribing course. However, local practices will dictate which route is most applicable.

Electronic prescribing

There has been a clear statement of intent that all chemotherapy medicines should be prescribed on electronic systems (NHS England 2014b). However, if electronic systems are unavailable, then preprinted proformas should be developed. No such edict applies to supportive therapies, though electronic prescribing is regarded as best practice. Prior to the most recent chemotherapy standards being published, it was clear the first cycle of any chemotherapy regimen should be prescribed by the consultant oncologist or haematologist (DOH 2014). This was a clear safety issue to ensure the treatment pathway is planned by a consultant, allowing for any amendments to the standard regimen based on the patients' fitness to receive chemotherapy, including adjustments for comorbidities. However, the most recent measures have adjusted this standard to say that named personnel with competence can prescribe the first cycle (DOH 2011, NHS England 2014). This means that competent NMPs can legitimately prescribe the first cycle of chemotherapy.

Training requirements

The training requirements for becoming an NMP are set out in the NMC document 'Standards of proficiency for nurse and midwife prescribers' (NMC 2015). Training is within higher education facilities and the curriculum is theory and practice based. It is designed to ensure proficiency in:

- Assessing a patient/client's clinical condition
- Undertaking a thorough history, including medical history and medication history, and diagnosing where necessary, including over-the-counter medicines and complementary therapies
- Deciding on management of presenting condition and whether or not to prescribe
- Identifying appropriate products if medication is required
- Advising the patient/client on effects and risks
- Prescribing if the patient/client agrees
- Monitoring the response to medication and lifestyle advice. (NMC 2014)

Supporting the training standards is a clear practice document – a single-competency framework for all prescribers, which is published by the National Prescribing

Centre (NPC 2012). This document is designed for all practitioners, including medical staff.

The quality of the NMP education programmes has recently been evaluated in a national survey (Smith et al. 2014). The survey results are reassuring in that almost 1,000 independent prescribers found the standards of training to adequately prepare individuals for practice.

Having a new prescribing skill is of course important, but there may be barriers within organisations to actually prescribe in practice (Farrell 2014). In supporting nurses to develop nurse-led clinics/service, the United Kingdom Oncology Nursing Society have produced a position statement to help practitioners plan and develop their contribution to care (Lennan et al. 2012). This statement suggests that the ability to prescribe is a gold standard rather than necessity, but it makes the case that a maturing and advancing profession should own nursing practice and not rely on the medical profession. It further outlines a framework for developing clinical services.

Audit and continuing professional development

Once qualified, it is important to remember that though an individual might have expertise in a speciality, they are a novice prescriber. The training course will demonstrate competence, but building confidence takes longer and requires ongoing support. With such an important skill, keeping up to date is key. Managers should be keen to understand prescribing activity, and the prescriber will need to demonstrate continuing professional development (CPD). In acute care settings, audit trails might be difficult to track all paper prescriptions across different operational systems. The practitioner may therefore find it easier to audit their own practice. However prescribing in the community will generate an automatic audit trail, and NMPs should access this information regularly from prescribing leads with area teams.

Demonstrating CPD can sometimes also be challenging, however there are lots of opportunities to reflect and learn. Some examples within practice might include MDT discussions, debates with pharmacists, reflecting on patient outcomes, discussions with GPs, managing side effects, meeting with representatives or updating policies. More formal examples include attendance at conference, reviewing NICE appraisals, or attending education days, journal clubs or university modules.

In demonstrating CPD and activity during appraisals, Pearce and Winter (2014) found that practitioners were often managed by non-prescribers, making assessment and reflection difficult. This team have developed a checklist to help managers understand prescribing practices and also provide guidance for the practitioner in how to relay practice and reassure the manager. The checklist is simple and covers:

- Is the NMP actively prescribing and is it relevant to role?
- Is the prescriber clear about their scope of prescribing and able to demonstrate up-to-date clinical, pharmacological and pharmaceutical knowledge relevant to their own area of practice?

- Is the prescriber able to discuss in context of prescribing, diagnosis and management options for the patient and follow up?
- Are they able to access the intranet NMP site?
- Do they know whom to make contact with for enquiry? (NMP administrator/ NMP lead)
- Has the NMP completed the relevant Trust paper work to comply with governance arrangements?
- Specific training/CPD is identified at appraisal to comply with policy.
- Has the prescriber been given time to comply with CPD requirements?
- Does the prescriber have a named supervisor?
- If relevant, has the NMP completed any intention to prescribe controlled drugs and returned it to the NMP administrator? (Pearce and Winter 2014)

This framework will ensure that dialogue is meaningful and facilitates a platform for safe prescribing for the prescriber and the organisation.

Conclusion

The NMP is here to stay and will become an increasingly important skill for nurses. Next year should see the results of a Cochrane review (Weeks et al. 2014). This much-needed review will assess the clinical, economic and humanistic health outcomes of non-medical prescribing for managing acute and chronic health conditions in primary and secondary care settings compared with medical prescribing. However it is likely to recommend the need to develop further robust research studies to increase the evidence base. As a profession, nurses need to embrace the skill and own the services they provide. However, they should never work in isolation and must remain connected with the MDT. Evidence confirms this is acceptable to patients, medical staff and the nurses themselves.

History tells us that nurses are curious; NMP has opened a new door; the new paths are wide and long; take the first step. . . .

References and further readings

Avery G, Todd J, Green G, & Sains K. (2007). Non-medical prescribing: the doctor nurse relationship revisited. *Nurse Prescribing*. 5: 109–113.

Baird A. (2001). Diagnosis and prescribing: the impact of nurse prescribing on professional roles. *Primary Health Care*. 11: 24–26.

Baird A. (2005). Independent and supplementary prescribing and PGDs. *Nursing Standard*. 19(51): 51–56.

Basford L. (2003). Maintaining nurse prescribing competences: experiences and challenges. *Nurse Prescribing*. 1(1): 40–45.

Berry D, Courtenay M, Bersellini E. (2006). Attitudes towards, and information needs in relation to, supplementary nurse prescribing in the UK: an empirical study. *Journal of Clinical Nursing*. 15: 22–28.

BMA. (2008). BMA calls for urgent meeting with Patricia Hewitt on plans to extend prescribing powers. (Press release 10th November 2005).

Bowden E, Horne N. (2011). A joint non-medical prescribing clinic for the management of patients requiring tyrosine kinase. Posters, 9th Annual BTOG Conference, Dublin, January.

Bradley E, Campbell P, Nolan P. (2005). Nurse prescribers: who are they and how do they perceive their role? *Journal of Advanced Nursing*. 51(5): 439–448.

Bradley E, Nolan P. (2007). Impact of nurse prescribing: a qualitative study. *Journal of Advanced Nursing*. 59(2): 120–128.

Brooks D, Rashid C, Kilty L, Maggs C. (2001a). Nurse prescribing. What do patients think? *Nursing Standard*. 17: 33–38.

Brooks D, Otway C, Rashid C, Kilty E, Maggs C. (2001b). The patient's view: the benefits and limitations of nurse prescribing. *British Journal of Community Nursing*. 6(7): 342–238.

Buckley P, Grime J, Blenkinsopp A. (2006). Inter and intra professional perspectives on non- medical prescribing in an NHS Trust. *The Pharmaceutical Journal*. 277: 394–398.

Clegg, A. (2006). Reflection on nurse independent prescribing in the hospital setting. *Nursing Standard*. 21(12): 35–38.

Cooper R, Anderson C, Avery T, Bissell P, Guillaume L, Hutchinson A, Lymn J, Murphy E, Ratcliffe J, Ward P. (2008). Stakeholders' views of UK nurse and pharmacist supplementary prescribing. *Journal of Health Service Research Policy*. 13(4): 215–221.

Courtenay M, Carey N. (2007). Preparing nurses to prescribe medicines for patients with diabetes: a national questionnaire survey. *Journal of Advanced Nursing*. 61(4): 403–412.

Courtenay M, Carey N, Burke, J. (2007). Independent extended nurse prescribing for patients with skin conditions: a national questionnaire. *Journal of Clinical Nursing*. 16: 1247–1255.

Courtenay M, Berry D. (2007). Comparing nurses' and doctors' views of nurse prescribing: a questionnaire survey. *Nurse Prescribing*. 5(5): 205–210.

Courtenay M. (2008). Nurse prescribing, policy, practice and evidence base. *British Journal of Community Nursing*. 13(12): 563–566.

Crew S. (2010). Non-medical prescribing in secondary care: an audit. *Nurse Prescribing*. 8(10): 498–502.

Day M. (2005). UK doctors protest at extension of nurses' prescribing power. *British Medical Journal*. 331: 1159.

Day M. (2008). Industry's push to woo nurse prescribers has been at "expense of nursing integrity". *British Medical Journal*. 336: 352.

Department of Health and Social Security. (1986). *Neighbouring nursing: a focus for care (Cumberlege report)*. London, Her Majesty's Stationery Office.

Department of Health. (1999a). *Making a difference*. London, HMSO.

Department of Health. (1999b). *Review of prescribing, supply and administration of medicines. Final report*. London, HMSO.

Department of Health. (2000a). *The Nursing Contribution to Cancer Care*. London, HMSO.

Department of Health. (2000b). *Consultation on proposals to extend nurse prescribing*. London, HMSO.

Department of Health. (2000c). *The NHS Cancer Plan*. London, HMSO.

Department of Health publications and statistics online. (2001). *Patients get quicker access to medicines*. http://webarchive.nationalarchives.gov.uk/+/www.dh.gov.uk/en/Publicationsandstatistics/Pressreleases/DH_4010748 [accessed 29.05.2015].

Department of Health. (2003a). *Supplementary prescribing by nurses and pharmacists within the NHS in England: a guide to implementation*. London, HMSO.

Department of Health. (2003b). *Nurse prescribers' extended formulary: Proposals to extend the range of prescription only medicines—Consultation.* London, HMSO.

Department of Health. (2004). *Nurse prescribing training and preparation: extended formulary prescribing and supplementary prescribing.* London, HMSO.

Department of Health. (2006). *Improving patients' access to medicines: a guide to implementing nurse and pharmacist independent prescribing within the NHS in England.* 1–68. London, HMSO.

Department of Health. (2007). *The cancer reform strategy.* London, HMSO.

Department of Health. (2009). *Chemotherapy services in England, ensuring quality and safety: a report from the National Chemotherapy Advisory Group.* London, HMSO.

Department of Health. (2011). *Manual for cancer services chemotherapy measures.* London, HMSO.

Department of Health. (2013). *Living with and beyond cancer: taking action to improve outcomes (an update to the 2010 The National Cancer Survivorship Initiative Vision).* London, HMSO.

DH. (2001). Patients to get quicker access to medicines. Department of Health. http://webarchive.nationalarchives.gov.uk/+/www.dh.gov.uk/en/Publicationsandstatistics/Pressreleases/DH_4010748 [last accessed 29.07.2015].

DH. (2002). More prescribing power for NHS nurses. Department of Health. http://webarchive.nationalarchives.gov.uk/+/www.dh.gov.uk/en/Publicationsandstatistics/Pressreleases/DH_4013072 [last accessed 29.07.2015].

Earwicker S. (2005). Extended prescribing by UK nurses and pharmacist : computer systems need to incorporate nurse prescribing. *British Medical Journal.* 331: 1337.

Farrell C. (2014). *An exploration of oncology specialist nurses' roles in nurse-led chemotherapy clinics.* Unpublished PhD thesis. University of Manchester.

Fitzpatrick M, Honnet R, Wall, A. (2008). Hospital inpatient perspectives on supplementary and independent prescribing by pharmacists. *Pharmacy Today.* 24(2): 19–25.

Fitzsimmons D, Hawker S, Simmond P, George S, Johnson C, Corner J. (2005). Nurse led models of chemotherapy care: mixed economy or nurse-doctor substitution. *Journal of Advanced Nursing.* 50(3): 245–252.

Gerard K, Tinelli M, Latter S, Smith A, Blenkinsopp A. (2014). Patients' valuation of the prescribing nurse in primary care: a discrete choice experiment. *Health Expectations* http://eprints.soton.ac.uk/364794/

Goswell N, Siefers R. (2009). Experiences of ward-based nurse prescribers in an acute ward setting. *British Journal of Nursing.* 18(1): 34–37.

Green B, Courtenay M. (2008). Evaluating the investment: a survey on non-medical prescribing. *Mental Health Practice.* 12(1): 28–32.

Griffiths P, Richardson A, Blackwell R. (2009). *Nurse Sensitive Outcomes & Indicators in Ambulatory Chemotherapy* London, National Nursing Research Unit.

Hall J, Cantrill J, Noyce P. (2006). Why don't trained community nurse prescribers prescribe? *Issues in Clinical Nursing.* 15: 403–412.

Hawkes B. (2005). *BMA calls for urgent meeting with Patricia Hewitt on plans to extend prescribing powers.* London, BMA.

Hay A, Bradley E. (2004). Supplementary nurse prescribing. *Nursing Standard.* 18(4): 33–39.

Holland et al. (2014). *Audit to show the role of independent non-medical prescribing in patients with lung cancer.* Kettering General Poster abstracts, 12th Annual British Thoracic Oncology Group Conference, London, December.

Home Office. (2012). *Circular: nurse and provisions pharmacist independent prescribing for Schedule 4 Part II drugs*, 16 April 2012. London, DH.

Humphries JL, Green E. (2000). Nurse prescribers: infrastructures required to support their role. *Nursing Standard*. 14: 35–39.

Jones K. (2009). Developing a prescribing role for acute care nurses. *Nursing Management*. 16(7): 24–28.

Jones K. (2011). The effectiveness of nurse prescribing. *Nursing Times*. 107 (26): 18–19.

Latter S, Courtenay M. (2005). Effectiveness of nurse prescribing: a review of the literature. *Journal of Clinical Nursing*. 13: 26–32.

Latter S, Maben J, Myall M, Courtenay M, Young A, Dunn N. (2005). *An evaluation of extended formulary independent nurse prescribing: executive summary of final report*. Southampton, University of Southampton.

Latter S, Blenkinsopp A. (2011). Non-medical prescribing: current and future contribution of pharmacists and nurses International. *Journal of Pharmacy Practice*. 19: 381–382.

Lennan E, Vidall C, Roe H, Jones P, Smith J, Farrell C. (2012). Best practice in nurse-led chemotherapy review. A position statement from UKONS. *Ecancer Medical Science*. 6263 doi: 10.3332/ecancer.2012.263.

Lennan E. (2014). Non-medical prescribing of chemotherapy: engaging stakeholders to maximise success? *Ecancer Medical Science*. 8: 417.

Lewis-Evans A, Jester R. (2004). Nurse prescribers' experiences of prescribing. *Journal of Clinical Nursing*. 13: 796–805.

Luker K, Austin L, Wilcock J, Ferguson B, Smith K. (1997). Nurses and GPs' views of the nurse prescribers formulary. *Nursing Standard*. 11(22): 33–38.

Luker K, Austin L, Hogg C, Ferguson B, Smith K. (1998). Nurse patient relationships: the context of nurse prescribers formulary. *Journal of Clinical Nursing*. 13: 26–32.

National Prescribing Centre. (2012). *A single competency framework for all prescribers* Liverpool, National Prescribing Centre.

NHS England. (2014a). *Manual for Cancer Services Chemotherapy Measures*. London, HMSO.

NHS England. (2014b). B15/S/a 2013/14 *NHS standard contract for cancer chemotherapy (adult)*. London, HMSO.

Nursing and Midwifery Council. (2006a). *Nurse prescribing and the supply and administration of medication. Position statement*. 2006.

Nursing and Midwifery Council. (2006b). Standards of proficiency for nurse and midwife prescribers. www.nmc.uk.org [accessed November 2014].

Nursing and Midwifery Council. (2014). *Effective practitioners by qualification, Communications department*. London, NMC.

Nursing and Midwifery Council. (2015). Standards of proficiency for nurse and midwife prescribers. http://www.nmc.org.uk/globalassets/sitedocuments/standards/nmcstandards ofproficiencyfornurseandmidwifeprescribers.pdf [accessed 29.05.2012].

Oliver A. (2002). *Cancer Services Collaborative Chemotherapy project*. Unpublished work.

Otway C. (2002). The development needs of nurse prescribers. *Nursing Standard*. 16: 33–38.

Pearce R, Winter H. (2014). Review of non-medical prescribing among acute and community staff. Nursing Management. 20(10): 22–26.

Poonawala YKS, Grahem-Clarke E. (2007). An audit of supplementary prescribing practice in an intensive care unit shows pharmacists can reduce the prescribing workload. *Pharmacy in Practice*. 17(7): 238–242.

Richmond S. (2005). Extended prescribing by UK nurses and pharmacists: triumph of common sense. *British Medical Journal.* 331: 1337.

Ryan-Woolley B, McHugh G, Luker K. (2007). Prescribing by specialist nurses in cancer and palliative care: results of a national survey. *Palliative Medicine.* 21: 273–277.

Salvage J. (2006). Nurses get a tongue lashing. *British Medical Journal.* 333: 265.

Scrafton J, McKinnon J, Kane R. (2012). Exploring nurses' experiences of prescribing in secondary care: informing future education and practice. *Journal of Clinical Nursing.* 21: 2044–2053.

Smith A, Latter S, Blenkinsopp A. (2014). Safety and quality of independent prescribing: a national survey of experience of education, continuing professional development clinical governance. *Journal of Advanced Nursing.* 70 (11): 2506–2517.

Stenner K, Carey N, Courtenay M. (2012). Prescribing for pain - how do nurses contribute? A national questionnaire survey. *Journal of Clinical Nursing.* 21 (23–24): 3335–3345.

Weeks G, George J, Maclure K, Stewart D. (2014). Non-medical prescribing versus medical prescribing for acute and chronic disease management in primary and secondary care. *Cochrane Database of Systematic Reviews*, Issue 7. Art. No.: CD011227. doi:10.1002/14651858.CD011227.

Chapter 6

Compassionate and effective communication

Key skills and principles

Alison Franklin, Claire Green, Nicola Schofield

Introduction

Communication skills are key to every area of healthcare. Effective communication is what enables us to establish the patient's agenda, i.e. perception, concerns, needs and expectations, adequately convey a sense of care and compassion, tailor information appropriately, negotiate involvement in decision-making and promote adherence to treatment and lifestyle changes (Weisman and Worden 1977, Harrison et al. 1994, Parle et al. 1996, Stewart 1996, Maguire and Pitceathly 2002, Farrell et al. 2005).

This chapter is based on an assumption that the vast majority of healthcare professionals would want nothing less than to be experienced by their patients as communicating compassionately and effectively. However for a variety of reasons and despite the best intentions of most healthcare professionals, communication difficulties and lack of emotional support continue to be highlighted as a problem for significant numbers of patients.

How well prepared are senior nurses to manage difficult or distressing conversations?

> Experience does not gather, merely with the passage of time but rather through a clinical dialogue with theory in which existing ideas, theory and past experience are challenged or confirmed.
>
> (Benner 1984, p36)

As nurses gain experience and seniority, there is an expectation that they will handle increasingly difficult and complex communication with patients and colleagues (NICE 2004, Department of Health 2004). However, this expectation has historically existed alongside an assumption that communication skills are innate and/or develop with experience.

Experience may well be a good teacher but communication does not reliably improve with experience *alone*. Rather it is a skill set that needs to be taught and developed, as in any other area of practice (Cantwell and Ramirez 1997, Maguire 1999). Nurses regularly report having received minimal communication skills training preregistration and feeling inadequately prepared to talk with patients about more complex and emotive issues such as life-changing illness, death and dying (Hjorleifsdottir and Carter 2000, Barclay et al. 2003). Small wonder, then, that lack of confidence and insufficient training in communication skills has been recognised as a significant source of workplace stress and burnout in healthcare professionals (Ramirez et al. 1996, Heaven et al. 2006).

This chapter invites the reader, whatever their current level of training and experience, to reflect on the topics listed below in relation to their own practice in order to affirm, challenge and build on existing skills and knowledge to increase confidence in communicating with patients and families in both every day and complex situations.

Topics for reflection

1. The importance of communication skills and the impact of communication on patients' physical and emotional well-being
2. The challenge of working with patients' emotions
3. Skills and strategies for effective communication

   - Empathy: a core clinical skill
   - Facilitative communication skills and behaviours
   - Using a patient-centred interview structure

4. Tips for personal survival

I. The importance of communication skills and the impact of communication on patients' physical and emotional well-being

Distress, anxiety and depression.

Cancer is a serious and potentially life-limiting disease. The surgery and treatment can be disfiguring and extremely unpleasant and can negatively impact on many areas of a person's life.

Numerous studies have reported that patients find the emotional aspects of dealing with cancer as difficult if not more difficult than the physical aspects, but they often feel unsupported in this area and unsure of where to get help (Macmillan 2006). The distress and worry caused by dealing with cancer can also lead to significantly increased risk of a clinical anxiety and/or depression in both the short and long term, as shown in Table 6.1.

Table 6.1 Risk of developing an affective disorder (anxiety and/or depression) (Massie 2004, Pitceathly et al. 2004, Mitchell et al. 2013)

	General population	Cancer patients	Carers/partners
Overall prevalence	12%	35%	33%

Are high levels of emotional distress inevitable?

International research dating back from the 1970s has consistently demonstrated that communication between healthcare professional and patient can impact significantly on psychological adjustment, satisfaction, adherence to treatment and quality of life in both the short and longer term (Stewart 1996, Street et al. 2009). Continuing high levels of distress including anxiety and depression are therefore not inevitable and there is evidence that the risk can be substantially reduced by supportive, effective communication and recognition and appropriate response to psychological needs. Sequential analysis of communication behaviours in interactions between healthcare professionals and patients has helped to identify problems in communication behaviours that impact on adjustment and coping, as shown in Table 6.2.

Risks in communication

The key communication tasks that form part of the overall consultation and illustrated in Table 6.2 are to some extent interdependent. Communication failures in one area will therefore compound the risk of failure in others.

When the patient's perception and concerns are not fully established

In busy clinics there can be a tendency for clinicians to recap their own understanding based on previous meetings or what is written in the notes, seek confirmation from the patient and then move on to give information.

> *So, Mrs Jones, you had your surgery and when you saw Mr Brown last week you were recovering nicely from that, I understand you have come today to talk about the next stage of treatment, is that right?'*

Alternatively, the patient's perception is often sought by asking, 'what have you been told?' Whilst this may reveal some of the patient's understanding, unfortunately disclosure is likely to be limited to a regurgitation of what has been said. The risk with both of these approaches to eliciting perception is that they do not uncover what the patient has *understood* and gaps or misperceptions in the patient's understanding of their situation may not be revealed. Neither are they likely to establish what has been the *emotional impact* of this (i.e. what concerns and fears have been raised).

Without knowing the patient's current level of understanding and their concerns it will be impossible to tailor information to the individual's needs and priorities. Furthermore, the continuing high level of distress and preoccupation with concerns will impede the patient's ability to process and recall the information that *is* given. The patient is therefore unable to fully participate in the decision-making process because they do not have sufficient relevant information and because their decision-making ability is impeded by the continuing distress.

Table 6.2 Key communication tasks impacting on adjustment and coping

Communication task	Impact on adjustment/coping	What happens in consultations
Acknowledging and working with emotions	Builds rapport Elicits clinically relevant information Reduces stress and level of emotion Increases information recall Enhances decision-making ability (Harari et al. 2000, Lelorain et al. 2012, Sep et al. 2014)	Clinicians underestimate patient level of distress (Ford et al. 1994) Clinicians predominantly respond to informational cues (questions) rather than emotional cues (Butow et al. 1995, Kruijver et al. 2001) The majority of emotional cues are met with premature reassurance, information and other behaviours that prevent further expression or exploration of the emotion (Wilkinson 1991, Zimmermann et al. 2007)
Eliciting concerns	Number and severity of concerns both correlates with and predicts high levels of anxiety and depression (Weisman and Worden 1977, Harrison et al. 1994, Parle et al. 1996, Farrell et al. 2005)	Up to 80% of patient concerns are not identified by health professionals Up to 70% of patients do not have ANY of their top three concerns recognised (Farrell et al. 2005)
Tailoring information	Perceived satisfactory level of information (i.e. tailored to the individual's needs and concerns) is linked with better psychological adjustment, lower levels of anxiety and depression and better quality of life (Fallowfield et al. 1990, Butow et al. 1995, Schofield et al. 2003)	Information-giving tends to be formulaic and dictated by the biomedical agenda (Ford et al. 1996) Patients are given insufficient space to absorb and respond to information (Ford et al. 1996) The more information that is given the less the patient recalls (Jansen et al. 2010
Enabling shared decision-making	Participation in decision-making is linked to significantly higher overall quality of life (Hack et al. 2005)	Clinicians routinely fail to recognise patients' individual preferences and priorities in decision-making (Rothenbacher et al. 1997, Mulley et al. 2012) Patients feel excluded from participation by clinicians communication behaviours (Ford et al. 1996, Rothenbacher et al. 1997, Jansen et al. 2010, Mulley et al. 2012, Zhou et al. 2014).

KEY POINTS ON THE RELATIONSHIP BETWEEN COMMUNICATION, PATIENT CONCERNS AND PSYCHOLOGICAL ADJUSTMENT

- High levels of distress including anxiety and depression are not inevitable and can be significantly mitigated by compassionate and effective communication.
- *Fully* establishing the patient's perception is a prerequisite for tailoring information and sharing decision-making.
- Perception involves *both* the patient's understanding of their current and future condition, treatment *and* the emotional impact of this (concerns).
- We therefore need to enquire about what has the patient understood AND how has that left them feeling.

2. The challenge of working with patients' emotions

What stops patients from sharing their concerns?

Many barriers to effective communication have been identified, including patients' own reluctance to disclose their concerns, environmental factors such as privacy and time constraints and the belief of some professionals that emotional or psychological aspects of care are not part of their role. This section is in no way intended to dismiss the very real difficulties and constraints within which healthcare professionals work. Rather it seeks to explore the difficulties experienced in eliciting concerns, tailoring information, sharing decision-making and working with emotions when the intention is to do so. It illustrates that paradoxically, it is the very desire to help that often results in behaviours that impede communication.

Healthcare professionals may feel that a key reason for not identifying patient concerns is that patients are reluctant to disclose them. Certainly it is true that patients may worry that they may be judged, they may burden or distress the health professional or may view the professional as too busy or not the 'right' person to talk to (Maguire 1985b, Booth et al. 1996, Heaven and Maguire 1997). For these reasons patients have a tendency not to disclose concerns directly but rather hint at their concerns via cues.

Cues are verbal or nonverbal hints or statements of an unpleasant underlying emotion that would require clarification from the healthcare provider to detect the presence of an underlying concern (Butow et al. 2002, Del Piccolo et al. 2006).

Cues can be thought of as the way in which patients test the water to see whether the listener is interested in or able to handle their emotional distress or indeed to test their own ability to say out loud what has so far remained unspoken.

Concerns are unpleasant emotion plus content, i.e. what is causing it.

Therefore an expression of worry alone, 'it feels quite daunting,' is a cue; we only have the concern when we know what feels daunting and why

Because concerns are most often expressed via cues, eliciting patient concerns relies on the healthcare professional's ability to hear, identify and respond appropriately to cues.

However the research indicates that healthcare professionals have a tendency both to miss at least 50 per cent of cues and to behave in ways which block the patient from further disclosure (Zimmermann et al. 2007).

Why cues are missed

In an applied discipline, competence and expertise develops through a process in which the practitioner becomes increasingly able to interpret clinical situations and assess which aspects are important and which are irrelevant to long term care aims. As has been suggested by Mulley (2012), amongst others, healthcare professionals have a tendency to interpret 'relevance' from a biomedical or nursing perspective. This may mean that the more experienced the healthcare professional becomes, the more they may attune primarily to hints of problems which feel relevant to the diagnosis, treatment or care from their specialist clinical point of view and that other issues raised by the patient may be filtered out as irrelevant.

Blocking and distancing behaviours

Behaviours which inhibit the patient from expressing their emotions and disclosing their concerns are known as blocking and distancing behaviours. Research suggests that in interactions with patients at least half of healthcare professionals' responses to cues have a blocking function (Wilkinson 1991). Several reasons have been identified for this.

Self-protection

Recognising and responding to potentially strong emotions may raise feelings of anxiety and distress and/or inadequacy in the healthcare professional. Similarly, constant exposure to loss, grief and mortality may evoke actual or feared issues for self and loved ones. As a defence against these difficult feelings the healthcare professional may feel compelled to avoid areas that feel personally painful, threatening or which they feel they cannot 'fix' (Maguire 1985a, Rosenfield and Jones 2004).

'Protecting' the patient

Some of the reasons for steering away from patients' emotions centre on the misperception that expressing strong emotions may in some way be damaging for the patient. We may fear this will negatively impact on the relationship, raise unrealistic expectations and unleash difficulties we have neither the time nor the skills to deal with, leaving the patient more vulnerable and distressed (Maguire 1999). When faced with patients' worries and distress, healthcare professionals want, understandably, to respond in ways intended to convey care, reassure, inform and problem-solve in order to relieve the distress. Unfortunately many of these behaviours in actuality have the opposite effect, as illustrated below.

When the desire to help impedes communication

Jackie Evans is 37 years old. She received a breast cancer diagnosis six weeks ago. She has had surgery and is about to start chemotherapy. She has two young children is recently separated and self-employed as a hair dresser. She is meeting Sue, her chemotherapy nurse, for the first time. Jackie has a number of concerns that are causing her immense distress and worry. Like most patients she does not disclose all of these directly but rather hints at them by offering cues (expressions of unpleasant emotion) or by stating the concern without expanding on the reasons behind it. Tables 6.3 to 6.5 give three examples of the ways in which the cues and concerns Jackie discloses might be blocked even though the responses were *intended* to mitigate distress.

Table 6.3 Example one: premature advice and information

Concern:	I'm **dreading** the chemotherapy.
Response:	What would help it feel less scary?
	Would it help if I take you through what's going to happen?
Intention:	To make the treatment seem less daunting and to reduce the fear/ distress.
Risk:	Assuming you know what the problem is and trying to fix it without having fully explored the patient's perspective and concerns.
Impact:	Both the question and the offer of information is premature because it is offered without knowing exactly what it is that Jackie is frightened about. Jackie doesn't know at this stage what would help. She is too polite to say no to the offer of information, but because she is preoccupied with the real concern she doesn't hear most of the information she is given and remains frightened.
Undisclosed concern:	When Jackie's friend lost her hair through chemotherapy, her children were teased and bullied at school. She is worried this will happen to her children too.

Table 6.4 Example two: moving away from the emotion

Cue:	When I got my diagnosis I was **devastated.**
Responses:	And how do you feel now? (focus on now, not then) What did they tell you about your diagnosis? (focus on facts, not feelings) How are the children coping with it? (focus on a different person)
Intention:	There's no point talking about things that can't be changed. Moving away from the emotion and focussing on something more manageable will help reduce the level of distress.
Risk:	By steering her away from talking about her strong emotion, Sue gives the message that Jackie's devastation is not something she wants to hear about.
Impact:	She discusses her feelings about some of these issues with Sue but does not disclose her biggest concern, which is still causing her a huge amount of distress and worry.
Undisclosed concern:	Jackie's divorce has been really acrimonious and she worries her ex may take advantage of her illness. She is frightened she could lose the house and sole custody of the children.

Table 6.5 Example three: trying to 'fix' the distress

Concern:	My friend had problems with her arm after radiotherapy and had to give up hairdressing, what if that happens to me?
Responses:	**Normalising:** That's completely understandable; you're bound to be worried. **Reassurance:** Try not to worry; it may not be as bad as you think. **Advice/Information:** Try not to compare yourself, everyone reacts to treatment differently.
Intention:	To lessen or take away the distress
Risk:	Sue has responded sympathetically but without knowing what happened to Jackie's friend or what specifically Jackie is worried about.
Impact:	Jackie appreciates Sue's concern but doesn't see how she could possibly understand. If everyone gets upset maybe she shouldn't make a fuss. The reassurance is both premature and false. Jackie remains just as worried and distressed but feels she is being told not to feel like that. It seems that Sue just doesn't understand.
Undisclosed concern:	Her friend's cancer came back. Jackie is frightened the same will happen to her.

Even when the reason behind a particular concern has been revealed, there is a tendency to block further disclosure by minimising the distress or rushing to fix things.

As we can see from the examples in this section, some of the most common barriers to patients communicating their concerns, needs and priorities are the very behaviours that are intended to be helpful and motivated by a need to 'fix' problems and reduce distress.

KEY POINTS ON PATIENTS' CONCERNS AND COMMUNICATION BY HEALTHCARE PROFESSIONALS

- Patients tend to disclose concerns indirectly via cues.
- Healthcare professionals miss or block over 50 per cent of patient cues.
- Many of the behaviours that are intended to reduce distress actually have the effect of blocking the patient from discussing their feelings.

3. Skills and strategies for effective communication

There is an expectation that all senior cancer clinicians will be able to overcome communication barriers, recognise and respond compassionately to patients' distress, elicit concerns and offer interventions such as emotional support and problem-solving (NICE 2004). In this section we will discuss the key skills and principles underpinning effective and compassionate communication and the importance of using these purposefully and in the context of an interview structure. First we will discuss the concept of empathy, what it is and why it is so important.

Empathy: a core clinical skill

Empathy has long been recognised as crucial to patient-centred communication and satisfaction with care. There is evidence that empathising with thoughts and emotions reduces the intensity of feeling, enables cognitive processing, reduces stress and leaves patients feeling valued and understood (Harari et al. 2000, Sep et al. 2014). Empathic responding has also been shown to enable further disclosure of concerns and elicit clinically relevant information, and is associated with higher levels of patient satisfaction, increased retention of information, increased compliance and better health outcomes (Weng et al. 2011, Lelorain et al. 2012, Steinhausen et al. 2014).

The exact nature and purpose of empathy, how it differs from other qualities such as sympathy or compassion and how it is conveyed has been subject of debate. There is often an assumption that concern and compassion equate with empathy. However, as we have seen earlier in the chapter, much of the blocking and distancing behaviour employed by clinicians is motivated by compassion. However, without a good understanding of the patient's feelings and perspective, the healthcare professional's attempts to alleviate the distress by offering advice/information/reassurance are premature and counterproductive.

Contemporary literature on empathy suggests that it can be described in terms of skills, abilities and motivation encompassing the following dimensions (Kim et al. 2004, Goleman 2007, Neumann et al. 2009).

On this basis working empathically requires the motivation to hear the patient's perceptions, feelings and wishes, the skills to enable the patient to share these and the skills and ability to convey to the patient that their experience is heard and understood. Empathy can be viewed as the core clinical skill underpinning compassionate and effective communication.

Dimensions of empathy

Cognitive: The ability to recognise and understand the other person's perspective or point of view

Emotional: The ability to sense the emotions of the other person

Compassionate: Seeing the distress or predicament the other person is in and being motivated to want to help them

Verbalised: To be effective empathy has to be *heard* by the patient

---

'Give empathy words'

We have earlier highlighted that it is not enough to empathically understand the other person's thoughts and feelings, we need to convey our understanding of their thoughts and feelings back to the other person so that they *hear* that they have been listened to and that their thoughts and feelings have been understood. Empathy therefore needs to be verbalised. To be effective it is important that empathy is offered as accurately as possible and in a tentative way that allows the patient to agree, correct or expand. The following examples are based on a four-point empathy scale devised by Mearns and Thorne (2011).

Levels of empathic responding

A patient has just been told her chemotherapy isn't working. (Sobbing and shaking her head) 'I can't take it in, what does this mean for me now?'

Level 0 = blocking – no recognition or evidence of understanding
    'I'm afraid there's no more treatment, but don't worry, we won't abandon you and we'll make sure you're comfortable.'
Level 1 = minimal acknowledgement – partial understanding
    'I'm sorry, it's difficult, isn't it?' (partially acknowledges the patient's feelings but misses both the quality and the depth)
Level 2 = accurate empathy – captures expressed thoughts and feelings and reflects them back
    'I can see you're just devastated . . . and finding it hard to take in . . . you're wondering what this means for you now?' (space given)

> Level 3 = depth reflection – captures not only what is expressed but also what is implied
>
> 'This news has been just devastating for you . . . and you're really struggling to take it in . . . it sounds as though you might be quite frightened about what it means for your future . . . would that be right?' (space given)

Note of caution!

Avoid making statements such as 'I understand how you feel'. It is impossible to completely comprehend how another person experiences their situation and it risks evoking a reaction of 'no you don't!'

KEY POINTS ON EMPATHY

- Empathic listening involves the ability to suspend one's own agenda temporarily in order to listen and observe carefully what is being said, not said or implied. It involves looking and listening for emotions and perceptions.
- Empathic responding requires verbally acknowledging the emotion the patient is experiencing i.e. saying what you are seeing, hearing or sensing without judgement and checking you have heard and understood the patient's thoughts and emotions accurately.
- AFTER doing this, any help and/or information offered should be appropriate and sensitive to the perceptions, concerns and needs of the other person.

Facilitative communication skills and behaviours

The skills and behaviours shown in Table 6.6 are those generally recognised as those that help patients to share their concerns, needs and priorities, so that the practitioner can tailor information appropriately and to enable the patient's participation in decision-making in any consultation.

Working with patient cues

As we discussed earlier, patients have a tendency to hint at their concerns, needs and priorities via cues. Cues have been defined as hints or expressions of a negative emotion. Working with cues therefore is working with emotions. When facilitative skills are linked to the patient's emotions they are far more powerful

Table 6.6 Facilitative communication skills and behaviours

EMPATHY

Active listening
Attention, eye contact, giving space, pauses and silences.
Minimal prompts: nods, 'mm-hmm,' 'go on'

Exploring the patient's perspective		*Acknowledging the patient's perspective*	
Skill	*Description/Example*	*Skill*	*Description*
Open questions:	'How are you?'	Reflection:	Repeating key words or phrases
Open directive questions:	'How has that left you feeling?'	Paraphrasing:	Describing the patient's perspective in your own words to check understanding and demonstrate listening
Screening question:	'Is there something else?'		
Negotiation:	'I imagine you have all sorts of worries about this; could you bear to tell me about them?'		
Empathic educated guess (depth reflection):	'Would I be right in thinking the diagnosis came as real shock to you?'	Summary:	Repeating back key themes and issues from the patient's perspective and checking you have heard correctly

(Wilkinson 1991 and Maguire et al. 1996)

Table 6.7 Using facilitative skills to block or distance emotional cues

		Skill	*Impact*
Nurse	How are you?	Open question	
Patient	**Not so bad**, thanks. **I just don't understand** why **I feel so tired all the time** though. (**sounds worried**)		
Nurse	So you're tired all the time. What other problems are you having?	Reflection (minimal acknowledgement)	Focusses on the physical
Patient	**Just the tiredness**	Open question	Disclosure is limited to the physical concern

in enabling the patient to disclose. In fact the same skills can also be used to steer away from the patient's emotion and towards the biomedical or nursing agenda. Tables 6.7 and 6.8 show an example of how disclosure of concerns can

Table 6.8 Using facilitative skills to facilitate disclosure of further cues and concerns

		Skill	Impact
Nurse	How are you?	Open question	
Patient	**I'm not so bad**, thanks. **I just don't understand** why I feel so **tired all the time** though. (**sounds worried**)		
Nurse	You sound worried about being so tired, what thoughts have been going through your mind about it?	Depth reflection Open question	Focusses on the emotional impact of the tiredness
Patient	Well, I know it can be a side effect of the treatment **I can't help worrying that it means the cancer is back.**		A further concern about recurrence is disclosed

be either facilitated or blocked using the same skills (the cues are highlighted in bold).

As can be seen in this example, working with patient cues requires the ability first to recognise the cue and second to respond appropriately.

Recognising cues

Cues may be expressed verbally or non-verbally

Non-verbal cues

Crying, restlessness, sighing, frowning, withdrawal, negative body posture

Verbal cues

Hints/statements of feelings: 'I'm not sure', 'I was hoping', 'I'm OK, really', 'I'm worried'
Emphasis or metaphor: 'It was bloody awful', 'it's not a bed of roses'
Life events: 'It's cancer', 'he's lost his job'
Repetition of neutral statements: 'I live alone'
Physiological signs of distress: Sleep disturbance, agitation, anergia
Questions: 'What does this mean for me now?' 'What happens next?'

KEY POINTS ON FACILITATIVE SKILLS

- Facilitative skills need to be used in the context of patient cues
- Facilitative skills can be used to block disclosure of concerns
- Acknowledging and exploring emotional cues is crucial to eliciting patient concerns

A truly patient-centred approach therefore utilises empathy and facilitative skills to pick up the patient's cues, establish the patient's concerns and work with the patient's agenda.

Using a patient-centred interview structure

Clinicians may be concerned that working in a patient-centred way equates to giving up any control over the interview process with chaos ensuing! Not so. Having a purposeful interview structure is helpful to both healthcare professionals and patients, enhancing confidence, safety and ensuring everything is covered. Having a patient-centred approach does not mean abandoning the professional agenda (i.e. what we need to find out and what we need the patient to know), but that the professional agenda is held back until the patient agenda regarding their condition is fully established. There are a number of consultation models available, however what all have in common are the fundamental principles shown below.

Principles underpinning a patient-centred consultation structure

- Fully establishing patient's perceptions and concerns is crucial to understanding the needs and priorities that inform the patient's decision-making process (Mulley et al. 2012)
- Giving information inhibits disclosure of further cues and concerns (Zimmerman et al. 2003)

Evidence-based consultation models therefore advocate *gathering* all relevant information before *giving* information, advice or reassurance. However it is important that within the overall structure both gathering and giving phases remain flexible and responsive to the individual patient.

Figure 6.1 is an adaptation of the Calgary-Cambridge interview structure (Kurtz et al. 2003). In this adaptation, empathy and actively working with cues

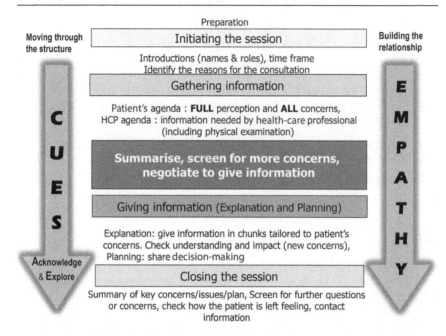

Figure 6.1 Interview structure adapted from Calgary-Cambridge (Kurtz et al. 2003)

and concerns are highlighted as the key behaviours that enable us to build the relationship, establish the patient's agenda, move through the interview at the patient's pace and maximise the chances that the information we give is appropriate, manageable and heard. The central framework offers a series of interview phases each with specific task and function that helps maintain purpose and optimise outcome.

The gathering phase

The purpose of this phase is to establish the patient agenda (perception, concerns, feelings and priorities) plus any additional information needed by the healthcare professional (HCP) to make an assessment or diagnosis. As we have earlier discussed in this chapter, for various reasons there is a tendency in healthcare professionals to shortcut this phase. This may involve selectively listening, focussing entirely on the physical, picking up cues related to the healthcare or biomedical agenda and avoiding or missing the patient's agenda. Where patient's emotions in the form of cues and/or concerns are disclosed, there is also a tendency to move prematurely to the explanation and planning phase, i.e. to reassure, try to deal with one thing at a time or attempting to preempt concerns by anticipating what information will be needed. This, as the evidence shows, inhibits the patient from disclosing further cues or concerns and compounds communication difficulties further on.

Time and effort invested in the gathering phase will ensure that the interview flows more smoothly in the giving phase because information can be tailored to the individual patient, and the patient is better able to listen to and retain information and participate in planning and decision-making.

Fully establish the patient's perception

As has been argued, patient perception is key to a patient-centred interaction. We cannot effectively tailor information and support until we have established what the patient knows, understands *and* feels about their situation. Questions for eliciting perception can be tailored for the context of the interview; for instance, in an interview where advanced care planning is being introduced, it would be useful to know what the patient's perception of their future health status is. Similarly, where treatment is being altered or withdrawn, establishing the patient's understanding of the purpose of the treatment, their perception of how it is working and any concerns about this is needed before the interview can move forward.

Strategies and skills for establishing perception:

Use open directive questions with a psychological focus

- What is your understanding of your condition?
- What are your thoughts?
- How do you see your future?
- How do you feel about how things are going so far?
- What did you understand about the purpose of the scan/tests/treatment?
- How has that left you feeling?

Work with the patient's cues

- You look anxious, is that right?
- Can you bear to tell me what is upsetting you?
- Can you tell me why that frightens you so much?
- You say you are hoping . . . you don't sound sure?

Establish the nature and extent of the patient's concerns

It is likely that the patient will have some concerns that cannot be 'fixed' by the health care professional (or anyone else), but it is still important to enable the patient to disclose these, because the mere expression of a concern is in itself helpful in mitigating distress and helping the patient to cope (Pennebaker 1993).

Resolution of concerns may be promoted by enabling the patient to generate her own solutions, or any offering relevant information, our own ideas and signposting or referral to appropriate sources of support. However it is essential that the cue and the underlying concern are explored *before* attempting to explore solutions, as illustrated earlier. This may require exploration at several levels. It is important to continue acknowledging what we are hearing throughout the consultation in order to demonstrate empathy and check understanding.

Often an empathic acknowledgement of the patient's cue alone will be sufficient encouragement to disclose the underlying concern. It is therefore important to allow a pause after empathising. This will enable the patient to agree or disagree, expand or clarify. Disclosure is also significantly enhanced by the use of open directive questions in response to cues. This can follow if needed. This process of empathising and exploring cues is illustrated below in a conversation with our patient Jackie and Sue her chemotherapy nurse. Cues are highlighted in bold, concerns disclosed are in italics.

Jackie: When I got my diagnosis I was **devastated**.

Nurse It sounds like it hit you very hard . . . PAUSE——— What was it that was particularly devastating for you? . . . PAUSE . . . empathy, open directive question

Jackie: I'm in the middle of a **really horrible divorce**, *I'm worried about coping with all the cancer treatment* and **everything else** as well

Nurse You're going through several horrible things at the same time and it feels quite overwhelming? Is that right? . . . PAUSE . . . you said you were worried about coping, could you bear to tell me what are some of the things you are having to cope with? reflection, empathy, negotiation to explore concern further

Jackie Well, my husband has been trying to get main custody of the children so he can have the house and *I'm really worried that he'll use my illness to say I can't look after them* . . . And *what if I can't look after them?* . . . My friend had breast cancer and she had to give up work, then it came back . . . she's been having treatment for years on and off, *I really worry that'll be me, and what impact that might have on my children, they're upset enough because of the divorce* . . . (**cries**)

Gather ALL concerns before giving

As we have earlier illustrated, the temptation as Jackie discloses her concerns may well be to begin offering advice or looking for solutions or to change the focus to the children and how they are coping. The risk in this is that it indicates to the patient that we are moving to the explanation and planning phase of the interview. As soon as we start giving advice or information or looking for solutions, the patient becomes far less likely to disclose further cues and concerns and the most difficult or important may remain undisclosed (Zimmerman et al. 2003). So rather than addressing each of Jackie's concerns one by one, it is really important that Sue actively elicits and acknowledges *all Jackie's concerns and screens for further concerns before moving to the explanation and planning phase of the interview.*

Nurse	I can see you're devastated . . . you're having to cope with a cancer diagnosis on top of the divorce . . . worried it will affect the outcome, the children and how it's going to affect them and also that things might turn out for you the way they did for your friend . . . is that about right? . . . PAUSE you said "everything" earlier, is there something else adding to the distress and worry?	Empathy Summary Reflection Screening question

The giving phase (explanation and planning)

What would help?

Remember that the mere expression of a concern is in itself helpful, so there may be no action required other than empathic acknowledgement. However if help or information is appropriate it is still important to ask the patient for their ideas before offering our own.

Tailoring information to the patient's concerns and needs

Identify what the person wants and needs to know
Obtain permission to give information
Give information in small chunks
Use clear and simple terms – jargon-free
Avoid detail unless requested
Use pauses – wait for a response
Allow information to sink in
Wait for a response
Check understanding and impact
  what has been understood?
  how is the patient left feeling?
  has the information raised new concerns?
Negotiate to continue
Deliver information at the patient's pace, not your own pace

Achieving the professional agenda within a patient-centred interview

A patient-centred interview is one which follows as its primary source the patient's agenda; i.e. it allows the patient's agenda to come first so that the patient's concerns and perception drive the information given and the care offered. This does not mean that the professional agenda is ignored. A focussed and proactive patient-centred approach will also help the patient to disclose clinically relevant information (Smith et al. 2011), which fully or semi covers the professional agenda too.

Earlier, a professional agenda was defined as

> The things that the professional wants to find out or needs to inform the patient of e.g. information essential for diagnosis, treatment or consent.

Where the interviewer needs further information in relation to a concern raised by the patient, for instance to assess the nature and extent of low mood or other symptoms, further exploration and clarification can follow after the patient's perception of the problem has been identified and acknowledged.

Other information not volunteered when exploring the patient's perception and concerns, but which the professional needs to know in order to arrive at a diagnosis or plan of care, can be kept to the end of the assessment or after the patient's concerns have been addressed at which point the healthcare professional can negotiate to ask for supplementary information and explain why it is needed. Similarly in the explanation and planning phase, any additional information that has not been specifically requested by the patient but needs to be given, e.g. for consent, ideally should be left until the end. Again there should be a negotiation to give further information, including why it is necessary.

We recognise that there are always exceptions to every rule, the important thing to bear in mind is that as much as possible, hold off on the professional agenda so that it does not overshadow or become more important than the patient's agenda.

KEY POINTS ON USING A PATIENT-CENTRED STRUCTURE

- Having a structure helps ensure that both patient and healthcare professional agendas are covered.
- Facilitative communication skills should be used to acknowledge and explore the patient's cues and concerns in all phases of the interview to keep the interaction patient-centred and at the patient's pace.
- Make sure to gather FULL perception and ALL concerns; summarise and screen for more concerns before giving (explanation and planning).
- Put the patient agenda before the professional agenda.

Identifying patients who may already be experiencing clinical anxiety and/or depression and referral for appropriate treatment

Throughout this chapter we have suggested that nurses are significantly placed to mitigate the risk of anxiety and depression in cancer patients by eliciting concerns, tailoring information and enabling shared decision-making through empathic patient-centred communication. Nevertheless there will still be a minority of patients at risk of affective disorder, for instance where there is a previous history of mental ill health (Parle et al. 1996). However, levels of anxiety and depression can be significantly reduced if recognised and appropriately treated (Sharpe et al. 2014, Walker et al. 2014).

Unfortunately, cancer clinicians fail to identify the majority of patients with probable anxiety or depression (Fallowfield et al. 2001, Lloyd-Williams and Payne 2002). When patients are recognised as depressed, fewer than half to one third are treated effectively (Sharpe et al. 2004, Walker et al. 2014). There is no expectation that oncology nurses should be able to diagnose or treat clinical depression and anxiety, but in order to make appropriate referrals they will need to be able to identify patients whose distress is at a level that may require specialist intervention (NICE 2004). This is important because when compared with patients receiving routine care, patients receiving an appropriate intervention for depression experienced a significant decrease in depression severity, anxiety, pain and fatigue and improvement in health functioning, quality of life and perception of quality of care (Sharpe et al. 2014, Walker et al. 2014). It is therefore helpful to be aware of the kind of criteria a mental health specialist would use.

Recognising clinical depression

The symptom is described as having the following qualities:

Key symptoms for clinical depression

Persistent low, sad or empty mood
and/or
Loss of interest, markedly diminished interest, lack of pleasure in, or inability to look forward to things

---

Mood cannot be lifted and is present most of the day nearly every day for a minimum of two consecutive weeks

Diminished interest in most or all activities, interests or things which is present most of the day nearly every day for a minimum of two consecutive weeks

Supporting symptoms (present for minimum of two consecutive weeks):

Weight Change – significant loss/gain when not dieting (or unexplained by treatment/illness) or decrease in appetite nearly every day.

Sleep disturbance – waking repeatedly or diurnal wakening (unexplained by physical illness), difficulty getting off to sleep or sleeping too much.

Psychomotor agitation or retardation – fidgety/restless, unable to sit still or being slower than normal. Nearly every day, observable by others or during interview.

Fatigue – loss of energy, feeling tired all the time, nearly every day.

Feelings of worthlessness/guilt – experiences these feelings nearly every day, which may be delusional and not merely self-reproach or guilt about illness.

Diminished ability to think – trouble in thinking or concentrating, difficulty in making decisions. This cannot be explained by a confusional state or medication.

Suicidal ideation – recurrent thoughts of death (not just fear of dying), recurrent suicidal ideation without specific plan, taken to the point of making plans or suicidal attempt.

Recognising an anxiety state

The symptom is described as having the following qualities:

Key symptoms

Excessive anxiety/worry, particularly nervous, anxious, a feeling of being on edge, unable to relax, tense, or a churning knot in the stomach, apprehensive expectation and/or anxious foreboding – which may or may not be related to current, past or future life events

---

The patient is persistently anxious or tense, or unable to relax for over 50 per cent of the time during the last four weeks.

The patient is unable to pull out of it.

This is a significant change from the patient's normal behaviour.

Diagnosis by a mental health specialist is dependent on the above symptom PLUS at least six of the supporting symptoms being present:

- Motor tension
- Vigilance & scanning
- Autonomic hyperactivity: tremble, twitch, shake

- Irritability
- Tense muscles, sore or achy
- Palpitations
- Impaired concentration
- Panic attacks
- Dry mouth
- Keyed up or on edge
- Difficulty in swallowing
- Nausea, vomiting

- Shortness of breath
- Difficulty in getting to or staying asleep
- Tire easily
- Sweating
- Intolerance of noise
- Frequency of micturition
- Dizziness
- Restless, can't sit still
- Diarrhoea

Depression may be mixed with anxiety. If you feel the patient has the key symptoms for either condition, and any of the supporting symptoms, consider referring on.

Introducing the idea of referring on

Summarise and agree the main concerns

Name the issues that may be more appropriately helped by another professional

'One of the things you mentioned is the way you have been feeling lately, your mood swings and irritability. Your mood problems sound as if they are affecting your life quite a bit? . . . I'd like to suggest that you talk to another member of the team, a colleague who specialises in working with mood problems and could help you more than I.'

Make clear who you are referring the person to: 'The person I am thinking of is Dr Lisa Jennings. She is a psychiatrist who works with the team here, and would be able to talk to you about what might help.'

Negotiate and check that the person is agrees to the referral: 'Is that OK? . . . I can see you are not very keen, but you know I think that Dr Jennings really is the best person to help you with this.'

---

4. Distress can be catching – tips for personal survival

Working in a patient-centred way has benefits for the healthcare professional. More accurate assessments, more satisfied patients and fewer complaints are all likely to increase job satisfaction and reduce stress; however working with patients' emotions can have an emotional cost for the healthcare professional. It is therefore important to be aware of and to accept our own strengths and weaknesses and to have strategies which make it possible to work with patient's emotional needs without becoming overwhelmed. These might include:

Personal refreshment

At work this could be as little as taking the 'scenic route' from one patient to the next, planning breaks and holidays, or taking time out.

Ensuring a good balance between work and home is also important; this might involve talking things through with friends and family or in doing social activities or hobbies you enjoy.

Work-based support

Share problems and successes with peers who understand and are in the same situation. Remember to share the good things too!

Prompt help in a crisis can make all the difference. Work at team building so that the support is there when you need it.

Review workload and professional development and support needs

Wherever possible:

> Review with your manager on a one-to-one level your own working practices, caseload and case mix to make sure your load is manageable.
> Access ongoing learning, study days, courses and reading.
> Supervision provides a place to reflect on work difficulties and helps identify learning needs as well as helping in solving them.

Have realistic expectations

Sometimes you or your relatives may have health issues. You may have been recently bereaved or experiencing a life crisis. At those times you may not feel able to manage the numbers or intensity of consultations you normally manage. There is nothing for you or your patient to gain if you 'soldier on' and become either totally depleted or feel you are mismanaging situations. It is more positive to talk to your colleagues or your manager and negotiate some protection of your workload until you feel ready to return to normal practice.

Conclusion

Communication skills have been identified as crucial in enabling patients to feel that they are treated with compassion, dignity and respect. Hopefully this chapter offers some ideas and skills to employ in your practice and more confidence that you can manage patient consultations effectively to meet your patient's needs and your own professional agenda. However whilst good communication skills give you greater potential to manage difficult interactions, it is worth keeping in mind that some situations are highly complex, and neither your communication skills nor your professional remit mean that you can be expected to manage every situation every time.

There is a vast difference between passing the buck, which usually means avoiding hearing the patients concerns, and a good referral on in which the patient's concerns have been identified and acknowledged before introducing the idea that another professional may be better placed to offer appropriate help.

Above all try to be as kind and compassionate to yourself as you would want to be with your patients.

> *'Compassion begins at home, and it is not how much we do but how much love we put in that action. Do not think that love has to be extraordinary. What we need is to love without getting tired.' (Mother Teresa, n.d.)*

References

Barclay, S, P. Wyatt, S. Shore, I. Finlay, G. Grande and Todd C. (2003). "Caring for the dying: how well prepared are general practitioners? A questionnaire study in Wales." *Palliative Medicine* 17(1): 27–39.

Benner, P. (1984). *From novice to expert.* Menlo Park, CA, Addison-Wesley.

Booth, K, P. Maguire, T. Butterworth T. and V. Hillier (1996). "Perceived professional support and the use of blocking behaviours by hospice nurses." *Journal of Advanced Nursing* 24: 522–527.

Butow, P.N., R.F. Brown, S. Cogar, M.H.N. Tattersall and S.M. Dunn (2002). "Oncologists' reactions to cancer patients' verbal cues." *Psycho-Oncology* 11(1): 47–58.

Butow, P.N., S.M. Dunn, M. Tattersall and Q. Jones (1995). "Computer based interaction analysis of the cancer consultation." *British Journal of Cancer* 71: 1115–1121.

Cantwell, B. and A. Ramirez (1997). "Doctor-patient communication: a study of junior house officers." *Medical Education* 31(1): 17–21.

Del Piccolo, L., C. Goss and S. Bergvik (2006). The fourth meeting of the Verona Network on Sequence Analysis "Consensus Finding on the appropriateness of provider responses to patient cues and concerns." *Patient Education and Counseling* 61(3): 473–475.

Department of Health (2004). The NHS Knowledge and Skills Framework (NHS KSF) and the Development Review Process. London, DOH.

Fallowfield, L., A. Hall, G. Maguire and M. Baum (1990). "Psychological outcomes of different treatment policies in women with early breast cancer outside a clinical trial." *British Medical Journal* 301: 575–580.

Fallowfield, L., D. Ratcliffe, V. Jenkins and J. Saul (2001). "Psychiatric morbidity and its recognition by doctors in patients with cancer." *British Journal of Cancer* 84(8): 1011–1015.

Farrell, C., C. Heaven, K. Beaver and P. Maguire (2005). "Identifying the concerns of women undergoing chemotherapy." *Patient Education and Counseling* 56(1): 72–77.

Ford, S., L. Fallowfield and S. Lewis (1994). "Can oncologists detect distress in their outpatients and how satisfied are they with their performance during bad news consultations?" *British Journal of Cancer* 70: 767–770.

Ford, S., L. Fallowfield and S. Lewis (1996). "Doctor-patient interactions in oncology." *Social Science & Medicine* 42(11): 1511–1519.

Goleman, D. (2007). Social Intelligence: The New Science of Human Relationships. London, Arrow Books.

Hack, T., L. Degner and P. Parker (2005). "The communication goals and needs of cancer patients: a review." *Psycho-Oncology* 14: 831–845.

Harari, A. S., Bookheimer SY and J. Mazziotta (2000). "Modulating emotional responses: effects of a neocortical network on the limbic system." *Neuroreport* 11: 43–48.

Harrison, J., P. Maguire, T. Ibbotson, R. Macleod and P. Hopwood (1994). "Concerns, Confiding and Psychiatric Disorder in Newly Diagnosed Cancer Patients: a Descriptive Study." *Psycho-Oncology* 3(3): 173–179.

Heaven, C., J. Clegg and P. Maguire (2006). "Transfer of communication skills from workshop to workplace: the impact of clinical supervision." *Patient Education and Counselling* 60: 313–325.

Heaven, C. and P. Maguire (1997). "Disclosure of concerns by hospice patients and their identification by nurses." *Palliative Medicine* 11(4): 283–290.

Hjorleifsdottir, E. and E. Carter (2000). "Communicating with terminally ill cancer patients and their families." *Nurse Education Today* 20: 646–653.

Jansen, J., J. van Weert, J. de Groot, S. van Dulmen, T. Heeren and J. Bensing (2010). "Emotional & information patient cues: the impact of nurses' responses on recall." *Patient Education and Counseling* 79: 218–224.

Kim, S., S. Kaplowitz and M. Johnstone (2004). "The effects of physician empathy on satisfaction and compliance." *Evaluation and the Health Professions* 27(3): 237–251.

Kruijver, I.P., A. Kerkstra, J.M. Bensing and H.B. van de Wiel (2001). "Communication skills of nurses during interactions with simulated cancer patients." *Journal of Advanced Nursing* 34(6): 772–779.

Kurtz, S., J. Silverman, J. Benson and J. Draper (2003). "Marrying content and process in clinical method teaching: enhancing the Calgary-Cambridge guides." *Academic Medicine* 78(8): 802–809.

Lelorain, S.A., A. Bredart and S. Sultan (2012). "A systematic review of the associations between empathy measures and patient outcomes in cancer care." *Psycho-Oncology* 21: 1255–1264.

Lloyd-Williams, M. and S. Payne (2002). "Nurse specialist assessment and management of palliative care patients who are depressed- a study of perceptions and attitudes." *Journal of Palliative Care* 18(4): 270–275.

Macmillan (2006). Worried Sick: The Emotional Impact of Cancer. London, Macmillan Cancer Support.

Maguire, P. (1985a). "Barriers to psychological care of the dying." *British Medical Journal* 291(6510): 1711–1713.

Maguire, P. (1985b). "Improving the detection of psychiatric problems in cancer patients." *Social Science and Medicine* 20(8): 819–823.

Maguire, P. (1999). "Improving communication with cancer patients." *European Journal of Cancer* 35(10): 1415–1422.

Maguire, P. and C. Pitceathly (2002). "Key communication skills and how to acquire them." *British Medical Journal* 325: 697–700.

Maguire P., Booth K., Elliott C., Jones B. (1996). Helping health professionals involved in cancer care acquire key interviewing skills—the impact of workshops. *European Journal of Cancer*. 32a:1486–1489.

Massie, M.J. (2004). "Prevalence of depression in patients with cancer." *Journal of National Cancer Institute Monographs* 32: 57–71.

Mearns, D. and B. Thorne (2011). Person-Centred Counselling in Action. London, Sage.

Mitchell, A., D. Ferguson, J. Gill, J. Paul and P. Symonds (2013). "Depression and anxiety in long-term cancer survivors compared with spouses and healthy controls: a systematic review and meta-analysis." *The Lancet* 14: 721–732.

Mother Teresa (n.d.). Centre for building a culture of empathy. http://cultureofempathy. com/references/Quotes/Compassion.htm#M [Last accessed 23.05.2015].

Mulley, A., C. Trimble and G. Elwyn (2012). Patients Preferences Matter: Stop the Silent Misdiagnosis. London, Kings Fund.

Neumann, M., J. M. Bensing, S. Mercer, N. Ernstmann, O. Ommen and N. Pfaff (2009). "Analyzing the nature and specific effectiveness of clinical empathy: a theoretical overview and contribution towards a theory-based research agenda." *Patient Education and Counseling* 74: 339–346.

NICE (2004). Guidance on Cancer Services: Improving Supportive and Palliative Care for Adults with Cancer. London, National Institute for Clinical Excellence.

Parle, M., B. Jones and P. Maguire (1996). "Maladaptive coping and affective disorders in cancer patients." *Psychological Medicine* 26: 735–744.

Pennebaker, J. (1993). "Putting stress into words: health, linguistic and therapeutic implications." *Behav. Res. Ther.* 31(6): 539–548.

Pitceathly, C., P. Maguire, P. Haddad and I. Fletcher (2004). "Prevalence of and Markers for Affective Disorders Among Cancer Patients' Caregivers." *Journal of Psychosocial Oncology* 22(3): 45–68.

Ramirez, A., J. Graham, M. Richards, A. Cull and W. Gregory (1996). "Mental health of hospital consultants: the effects of stress and satisfaction at work." *The Lancet* 347: 724–728.

Rosenfield, P. J. and L. Jones (2004). "Striking a balance: training medical students to provide empathetic care." *Medical Education* 38(9): 927–933.

Rothenbacher, D., M. P. Lutz and F. Porzsolt (1997). "Treatment decisions in palliative cancer care: patients' preferences for involvement and doctors' knowledge about it." *European Journal of Cancer* 33: 1184–1189.

Schofield, P., P. Butow, J. Thompson, M. Tattersall, L. Beeney and S. Dunn (2003). "Psychological responses of patients receiving a diagnosis of cancer." *Annals of Oncology* 14: 48–56.

Sep, M., L. van Osch, L. van Vliet, E. Smets and J. M. Bensing (2014). "The power of clinicians affective communication: how reassurance about non-abandonment can reduce physiological arousal and increase information recall in bad news consultations." *Patient Education and Counseling* 95: 45–52.

Sharpe, M., V. Strong, K. Allen, R. Rush, K. Postma, A. Tulloh, P. Maguire, A. House, A. Ramirez and A. Cull (2004). "Major depression in outpatients attending a regional cancer centre: screening and unmet treatment needs." *British Journal of Cancer* 90: 314–320.

Sharpe, M., J. Walker, C. Holm Hansen, P. Martin, S. Symeonides, C. Gourley, L. Wall, D. Weller and G. Murray (2014). "Integrated collaborative care for comorbid major depression in patients with cancer (SMaRT Oncology-2): a multicentre randomised controlled effectiveness trial." *The Lancet* 384 (9948): 1099–1108.

Smith, A., I. Juraskova, P. Butow, C. Miguel, A. Lopez, S. Chang, R. Brown and J. Bernhard (2011). "Sharing vs caring – the relative impact of sharing decisions versus managing emotions on patient outcomes." *Patient Education and Counseling* 82: 233–239.

Steinhausen, S., O. Ommen, S. Thum, R. Lefering, T. Koehler, E. Neufebauer and H. Pfaff (2014). "Physician empathy and subjective evaluation of medical treatment outcome in trauma surgery patients." *Patient Education and Counseling* 95: 53–60.

Stewart, M. (1996). "Effective physician-patient communication and health outcomes: a review." *Canadian Medical Association Journal* 152: 1423–1433.

Street, L., G. Makoul, N. Arora and R. Epstein (2009). "How does communication heal? Pathways linking clinician-patient communication to health outcomes." *Patient Education and Counseling* 74: 295–301.

Walker, J., C. Holm Hansen, P. Martin, S. Symeonides, R. Ramessur, G. Murray and M. Sharp (2014). "Prevalence, associations and adequacy of treatment of major depression in patients with cancer: a cross sectional analysis of routinely collected clinical data." *The Lancet Psychiatry* 1(5): 343–350.

Weisman, A. and J. Worden (1977). "The fallacy of post-mastectomy depression." *The American Journal of the Medical Sciences* 273(2): 169–175.

Weng, H., J. Steed, S. Yu, Y. Liu, C. Hsu, T. Yu and W. Chen (2011). "The effect of surgeon empathy and emotional intelligence on patient satisfaction." *Advances in Health Science Education* 16: 591–600.

Wilkinson, S. (1991). "Factors which influence how nurses communicate with cancer patients." *Journal of Advanced Nursing* 16: 677–688.

Zhou, Y., G. Humphris, N. Ghazali, S. Friderichs, D. Grosset and S. Rogers (2014). "How head and neck consultants manage patients' emotional distress during cancer follow-up consultations: a multilevel study." *European Archives of Otorhinolaryngol. European Archives of Oto-Rhono-Laryngology.* Doi: 10.1007/S00405.014-3209-x

Zimmerman, C., L. Del Piccolo and M. Mazzi (2003). "Patient cues and medical interviewing in general practice: examples of the application of sequential analysis." *UI* 12(2): 115–124.

Zimmermann, C., L. Del Piccolo and A. Finset (2007). "Cues and concerns by patients in medical consultations: a literature review." *Psychological Bulletin* 133(3): 438–463.

Chapter 7

Developing and evaluating nurse-led clinics

Carole Farrell

This chapter describes how nurse-led clinics have developed in the UK, summarising the key changes to legislation that have enabled nurses to lead services and develop nurse-led clinics. Implications for professional practice will be discussed, including education, training and clinical competence within nurse-led clinics. The different methods of assessing clinical competencies will be outlined, and consideration will be given to the merits of medical mentors, clinical supervision and systems of ongoing clinical appraisals. There will also be a step-by-step plan of how to set up a nurse-led clinic, including general points for consideration and tips for success. The importance of evaluation through audit and research will be discussed, including different methods that may be used.

Key policy influences

There are three main areas where policy and changes to legislation have influenced the development of nurses' roles and nurse-led clinics:

1. The reduction in junior doctors' hours forced the NHS to look at redesigning the workforce to meet the clinical needs of patients and provide appropriate clinical management to address the reduction in medical staff (Ferguson and Kearney 2000, DH 2007, 2008, 2009; NCAG 2009).
2. The nursing professional bodies (UKCC 1992, NMC 2008) made plans to allow nurses to extend their roles and take on some of the tasks that were previously within the doctors' domain. This revolutionised the scope of professional nursing practice and resulted in many nurses running clinics and services independent of medical staff.
3. The introduction, and later expansion, of non-medical prescribing has made has made fundamental improvements to enable nurses to provide more comprehensive and holistic packages of care for patients (DH 2006, Courtney et al. 2009, Stenner and Courtenay 2008a, 2008b).

Development of nurse-led clinics in the UK

Nurse-led clinics in the UK evolved from primary care, where practice nurses set up clinics for patients with chronic diseases such as diabetes (Clark et al. 2011), asthma (Clack 2009) and hypertension (Clark et al. 2011; Woodward et al. 2010; Chummun 2009). The later expansion within GP practices included nurse practitioners / advanced nurse practitioners and other health professionals, where nurses substituted for doctors and appeared to adopt a medical model of care. More recently in primary care there have also been an increasing number of district nurse clinics (Griffith and Tengnah 2013) and nurse-led clinics focusing on screening and risk assessments (Koelewijn-van Loon et al. 2009, Gulzar et al. 2007), which crosses the boundaries of work traditionally undertaken in secondary care.

Nationally nurse-led clinics are being undertaken for a wide variety of diseases and patient groups across secondary and tertiary care. This includes a pan-London nurse-led tuberculosis service (Belling et al. 2012), nurse-led genetics clinics (O'Shea et al. 2012), and a ward-based nurse-led clinic to manage postoperative problems after thoracic surgery (Williams et al. 2012). Some nurse-led clinics in secondary care have focused on chronic diseases such as coronary heart disease (Schadewaldt and Schultz 2011; Murchie et al. 2005; Raftery et al. 2005), rheumatology (Ndosi et al. 2011), diabetes (Mason et al. 2005; Youngman 2004) and epilepsy (Hadjikoutis and Smith 2005). However, nurse-led clinics are also built around patient pathways in order to reduce waiting times for patients (Lane and Minns 2010; Shakeel et al. 2008). The nature of nurse-led clinics in hospitals are diverse, and include nurse-led paediatric clinics to manage sensitive issues such as continence (Rogers 2008), sexually transmitted disease/HIV (Challenor et al. 2006), and sleep apnoea (Tomlinson and Gibson 2006); whilst other nurse-led clinics focus on one specialist area, such as dermatology (Duce and Gouldstone 2006; Moore et al. 2006).

Internationally there is variability in the number and nature of nurse-led clinics, which include continence, wound care (Shiu et al. 2012), diabetes (Edwall et al. 2008), rheumatology (Bala et al. 2012), hypertension (Kengne et al. 2009) and HIV/AIDS (Labhardt et al. 2009). However, the legislation in each country is variable and may restrict the development and expansion of nurses' roles and nurse-led clinics.

Nurse-led clinics in oncology

Within oncology there has been a rapid increase in the number and range of nurse-led clinics in the UK over the past ten years. Studies show increasing clinical demands to be one of the main drivers for nurse-led clinics (Allinson 2004). There are indications that clinics are exceeding capacity and medical staff feel overburdened (Anderson 2010, Turner and Wells 2012) with an increasing number of patients within medical clinics (James et al. 1994, Allinson 2004, Booker et al. 2004, Anderson 2010). There have also been reports of increasing waiting times for patients (Strand et al. 2011, Anderson 2010, Turner and Wells 2012), which is exacerbated by government targets placing pressure on clinical services, for example the need to see patients within two weeks of referral if cancer is suspected (Cox et al. 2006).

To address clinical demands. nurses, working in partnership with doctors, may select a group of patients that can be seen independently within a nurse-led clinic, thus easing the pressure (and numbers) within the medical clinic. However, focusing on patient numbers and medical workloads seems to give priority to a medical model of care focusing on doctor-nurse substitution, rather than patient-focused care using nursing values.

Ways of working in nurse-led clinics

Many nurses in nurse-led clinics will work to a protocol, which provides guidelines and role boundaries, often containing specific criteria to determine the type of patients they can see, and what they are allowed to do, including when to refer patients back to medical colleagues (Farrell 2014, Turner and Wells 2012, Strand et al. 2011, Jeyarajah et al. 2010, Macleod et al. 2007, Knowles et al. 2007). Protocols for nurse-led clinics that may be written purely by medical consultants can create restrictions in the scope of nurses' practice, therefore protocols written jointly by nurses and doctors will ensure that nurses' opinions are incorporated. Protocols can be used in a variety of settings to provide guidance for nurse-led clinics, including chemotherapy (Farrell 2014, Farrell and Lennan 2013) and radiotherapy (James et al. 1994). Similarly, written protocols can also guide the delivery of nurse-led telephone clinics (Anderson 2010, Beaver et al. 2009, Booker et al. 2004).

Other studies identify an assessment proforma designed by nurses, incorporating nursing assessments in addition to medical assessments, which may include a greater focus on psychological issues (Moore et al. 2006, Wells et al. 2008, Beaver et al. 2007). This suggests that there may be additional benefits for patients by amending the standard medical model of care and incorporating nursing elements.

In contrast, some nurse-led clinics are based primarily on patients' needs, with a nursing focus that offers an alternative model of care. For example, a randomised controlled trial comparing nurse-led and traditional medical management clearly identified the importance of nurses in undertaking comprehensive holistic patient assessments (Corner 2003, Moore et al. 1999, 2002). This increased understanding of key aspects of patients' experience that were not evident in standard medical follow-up. Similarly, Cox et al. (2008) demonstrated how complex and sensitive information and concerns can be explored using holistic assessments that include psychological, social, sexual and spiritual assessments.

Training

Few studies report what training nurses complete in order to undertake their extended role within nurse-led clinics. In the UK training may include clinical examination skills (Sheppard et al. 2009, Winter et al. 2011) and non-medical prescribing (Winter et al. 2011). The MSc in advanced nursing practice or

MSc in clinical nursing are well recognised as providing comprehensive university-accredited training for advanced nurse practitioners/nurse clinicians in the UK. However, academic institutions also offer modules or short courses on specific aspects of clinical examination, such as breast examination. In addition, many nurses undertake 'in house' clinical examination skills training, which is often based on 'shadowing' doctors (Moore et al. 1999, Sardell et al. 2000, Sheppard et al. 2009) or advanced nurse practitioners. This type of training relies solely on another health professional assessing nurses' competence to undertake clinical examination skills, or certain medical procedures, in their role as clinical/medical mentor. This generally involves assessing nurses' competence over a fixed period of time, and training may end when the nurse has completed a designated number of examinations or medical procedures. Whilst this type of training may be very good from a clinical perspective, there is no formal recognition of the training, which may create difficulties if nurses move to another hospital trust. The lack of standardisation with informal clinical training can also create local variations in the training undertaken and assessment of competencies.

There is also a lack of research evidence on clinical skills' training; Warren (2007) reports that nurses undertook three months supervised training with the lead cancer nurse and theoretical training on breaking bad news, however no details are given on the content of training and assessment of competencies. Training for non-UK nurses is only mentioned in two studies: a half-day session on telephone communication skills (Kimman et al. 2010) and six months training by a consultant surgeon on clinical examination and sigmoidoscopy (Strand et al. 2011).

Variability in clinical training for nurses and assessment of competencies creates uncertainties regarding individual nurses' professional practice, which may cause patients, other health professionals and the general public to question nurses' roles and responsibilities. Greater transparency and national standardisation is needed to address this, together with further research.

In addition to achieving competence with clinical skills and non-medical prescribing, it is important that nurses are able to maintain such skills over time; however this is generally not addressed. It is clear that nurses' confidence in their ability to undertake clinical examinations deteriorates over time when nurses use their skills infrequently (Farrell 2014). There are also examples where nurses have been training in clinical examination skills yet have not used their skills in clinical practice (Farrell 2014), which raises questions regarding the rationale for undertaking this type of training. The same is also true for non-medical prescribing, since there is evidence that nurses have undertaken training but do not prescribe in clinical practice (Farrell 2014). Therefore it is important to carefully consider what skills and training are actually needed for individual clinical roles, rather than simply gathering a skill set. Furthermore, the financial impact and impact on resources and services whilst nurses are undertaking training should be considered.

Types of nurse-led clinics in oncology

The majority of nurse-led clinics in oncology appear to be for routine follow-up after completion of adjuvant therapy; however current reductions in routine medical follow-up may lead to considerations of alternative methods of follow-up, such as telephone monitoring (Beaver et al. 2007). The reduction in junior doctors' hours has also created gaps in service provision for clinical/surgical assessments and procedures, therefore nurses have expanded their roles to undertake preoperative assessments and minor surgical procedures, such as taking biopsies, nipple tattooing, and central line insertion.

Value for money

One of the most fundamental aspects within the Cancer Reform Strategy is the need to ensure quality of care within service provision (DH 2007). However there is also a strong emphasis on providing 'value for money' within cancer service delivery, and this seems to have become one of the main local drivers for nurse-led services within NHS hospital trusts. Therefore it is important that issues of quality are not lost within this process. However if nurse-led services are set up as a substitute for medical management, it seems crucial to evaluate their effectiveness and acceptability to patients, including the identification of potential differences from patient's perspectives between nurse-led and medical management. This seems particularly important given that a further pledge from the Cancer Reform Strategy is to focus cancer spending on cost-effective interventions that make a difference to patients (DH 2007).

Setting up nurse-led clinics

Setting up a new nurse-led clinic will often take several months of preparation and organisation; however the time invested is well spent and will pay dividends in the success of the clinic.

The following step-by-step guide is not meant to be prescriptive, but to provide useful general tips on how to set up a new nurse-led clinic, and is based on years of experience in setting up and running nurse-led clinics in oncology.

1. *Planning*: It is important to have a clear plan or vision of how the clinic will run, setting out the type of patients, the remit and activities within the clinic, and considering the setting. Once you have a broad outline of the clinic it is essential to meet with other health professionals, including medical consultants, nurses and different managers to ensure your plans achieve consensus.
2. *Location*: Determining the location of your new clinic and obtaining a clinic space for a designated period of time may be one of the most challenging aspects of setting up a new nurse-led clinic. Traditionally medical consultants have priority over clinical space in outpatient departments, and capacity

---

10 Top Tips for Setting up Nurse-led Clinics

1. Careful planning takes several months but will pay dividends
2. Plan every aspect of your clinic step by step to identify potential issues
3. Carefully consider what training and skills you will need
4. Teamwork is crucial, avoid working in isolation where possible
5. Ensure support from colleagues: nursing, medical and administrative
6. Consider mentorship from a medical consultant
7. Consider clinical supervision from someone who understands your role
8. Organisation and timing are crucial to avoid patients' waiting
9. High quality documentation is vital in medical notes
10. Arrange appropriate cover and consider succession planning

---

levels can restrict the availability of clinic rooms, therefore early discussions with the manager who allocates clinic room is vital. Once you have a designated clinic room on a specific day and time, you can begin setting up your clinic. However, it is important to decide whether to set up your clinic within or parallel to a medical clinic so that colleagues are close at hand if medical advice is needed, or whether it can be independent from the rest of the clinical team.

3. *Support*: Obtaining support in setting up your nurse-led clinic is vital, and you need to involve a variety of people within the hospital. This can take time, but without good support and consultations with a wider team of people your clinic can rapidly fail. Successful nurse-led clinics rely on teamwork and collaboration, and nurses should try to avoid working in isolation.

- Medical consultants can make or break nurse-led clinics; therefore you need a clear plan of your aims. This includes explaining how the clinic will benefit patients and service delivery, including the impact on existing clinical services, discussing your role and activities within the clinic and protocols. Medical consultants are likely to want facts and figures about the number of patients you will see with the frequency and time for appointments. They will also need reassurance about your skills and competencies to achieve this, and you will need a written protocol outlining your scope of practice within the clinics, which should be signed by the consultant. This represents a written contract for your role within the clinic.

- Nurse managers can also influence the success of your clinic since they determine your job description and scope of practice, monitoring with annual appraisals. Lack of support from nurse managers can have a detrimental effect on your ability to undertake nurse-led clinics.

- Outpatient managers play a crucial role in the practical aspects of nurse-led clinics. It is important to gain their support for the smooth running of your clinic. Depending on the nature and location of your nurse-led clinic you may need a clinic nurse / healthcare support worker to assist you by guiding patients to and from the clinic room, bringing medical notes and other activities.
- The manager of health records / administration can provide vital support in ensuring the timely delivery of patients' notes for your clinic and may help with some secretarial support if needed. They can help you to decide what proformas you need for your clinic, such as written annotations/notes and appointment sheets. However there are likely to be differences in local organisations regarding such operational procedures. In addition you should discuss any procedures that need to be undertaken within your clinic, such as bloods, X-rays, scans and dressings, since they will need to be recorded and coded for financial purposes.
- Support from nursing colleagues is important to ensure that they understand the aims and objectives of your nurse-led clinic. In particular you should discuss how this will fit with their roles and determine role boundaries where roles are similar, or where your role is changing. Sometimes working out the boundaries can be complex but consensus is important to reduce any antagonism if a colleague feels that you are stepping on their toes.
- Support from other colleagues who may be involved in any aspect of your clinic will be helpful, for example receptionists, chemotherapy nurses, therapy radiographers, physiotherapists, dieticians. Again this will vary according to the nature of your clinic and local organisations/ availability.
- Support from patients and their family are vital, although this will be an ongoing process as your clinic continues. However, prior to setting up your clinic it is helpful to ask patients for their opinions, discussing what you plan to do and the potential benefits for them. This could be done informally by asking several patients open questions, or by developing a semistructured survey to obtain anonymous opinions from a larger number of patients, or formally by a feasibility research study.

4. *Organisation*: Good organisational skill is the key to successful nurse-led clinics, ensuring that clinics run smoothly and in a timely manner to avoid patients waiting unduly. Some of the operational aspects can be fine-tuned once the clinic is up and running, however it will be helpful to consider some aspects of this in the planning stages.

5. *Timing*: Timing is particularly important when determining the duration of appointments and the number of patients that you can realistically see within one clinic session. If you are taking on specific episodes of care, such as follow-up, chemotherapy or radiotherapy, you will need to assess the overall

number of patients that have been seen in the past month or three months in order to work out how many patients need to be seen within your clinic. In addition you need to consider whether the clinic can be overbooked, and if so by how many patients in one session.

6. *Consultation activities*: Carefully considering what you plan to do within your clinic will help to determine how much time you will need for each appointment and how many patients that you can realistically see in one session. It is important if you break this down into specific actions and develop your own structure for consultations. For example, consider history taking, including specific questions and verbal assessments, treatment discussions/ information, clinical examinations and prescribing, if required. These are traditional elements of medical consultations, therefore should be tailored to fit the requirements of your clinic.

   • Communication skills are important and should focus on identifying cues and eliciting patients' concerns as well as focusing on physical symptoms, treatment and information, and this will have a positive impact on patients (see Chapter 6). Some nurses report difficulties with 'closed door consultations' (Farrell 2014), therefore this may require some practice to build nurses' confidence, and mentorship or clinical supervision could be helpful.

   • Clinical examinations should be undertaken as necessary, rather than routine practice in some clinics where the potential benefit is minimal. If you do need to undertake regular clinical examinations, ensure that you have the competence and confidence for this. The time taken for clinical examination should also be taken into account when planning time for each appointment. However, if clinical examinations are very infrequent, you may need to consider whether referral to other health professionals, such as doctors, may be more appropriate. For example, many chemotherapy nurse-led clinics do not require clinical examinations to be undertaken.

   • The need for prescribing within nurse-led clinics should be determined in the planning stage. If you are not an independent prescriber you need to consider how you will arrange a prescription if patients need one. If you are an independent nurse prescriber you need to consider the range of medicines that you are likely to prescribe, and whether this falls within your area of experience and competence. This should also be discussed with your medical consultant/mentor, and may need to be outlined in your protocol. The majority of hospitals in the UK use electronic prescribing; therefore you need to allow additional time for this within your clinic. An increasing number of nurses now prescribe chemotherapy, although some areas still debate who can prescribe the first cycle of treatment. Although this can be prescribed after each consultation, some prefer to prescribe subsequent cycles of chemotherapy for all patients at the end of clinic, or indeed prescribe several cycles in advance.

7. *Documentation*: Each clinician has their own preference for making notes/ annotations of each consultation with patients, and nurses have the same options. Some will prefer to make hand written notes during or following each consultation, whilst others prefer to use a digital voice recorder, which is later transcribed. This should be undertaken by a medical secretary and recorded in a similar format to medical consultations. However, systems are changing with the introduction of electronic patient records, and some nurses directly input electronic notes after each consultation. This will vary according to local rules and operational processes.

8. *Unexpected events*: You also need to determine strategies for untoward events, such as patients attending your clinic when they are acutely unwell or have unexpected treatment toxicities, patients with severe psychological distress, if patients need referral to another health professional, or if you detect potential cancer recurrence. Considering all possibilities in the planning stages and discussing strategies with your medical consultant/mentor will facilitate timely actions within the clinic if such events occur. An outline of events and strategies should be incorporated into your protocol, since this represents the clinical guidelines for your clinic and determines your levels of responsibility and accountabilities.

9. *Post-clinic activities*: A nurse-led clinic does not finish once the last patient has been seen. There are several activities that are generally undertaken after completion of the clinic session, including:

- The safe removal/storage of patients' medical notes
- Ensuring that each patient has a follow-up appointment
- Ensuring that all necessary prescribing has been undertaken
- Letters, including consultation summaries to the patient's GP and other health professionals or possible referrals to other consultants. This often requires secretarial support; therefore liaison with the medical secretaries is crucial to ensure letters are sent in a timely manner.
- Further investigations may be required. This may be requested following individual consultations or after completion of the clinic. However the nurse may also be responsible for checking and interpreting the results, informing the patient and ensuring that appropriate action is taken. Strategies for this should be discussed with the medical consultant/mentor in the planning stages.

10. *Cover and succession planning*: Trying to operate a successful nurse-led clinic completely on your own is a very difficult task, since you cannot cover every week of the year due to annual leave and potential sickness. The success of a nurse-led clinic relies on continuity of high quality care, therefore you need to organise appropriate cover for the clinic in your absence, otherwise clinics will have to be cancelled and patients inconvenienced. Cover for nurse-led clinics may be another nurse with similar skills, experience and competencies, or a doctor, however this must be carefully negotiated in the

planning stages. Training a nurse in a more junior role within your nurse-led clinic can also help with career development and succession planning, however this can be considered further once the clinic is well established.

Clinical outcomes and nurse-led clinics

Wong and Chung (2006) suggest an important link between the processes of care within nurse-led clinics and the outcomes that nurses can achieve. Clinical outcomes may be defined as a change in the patient's health status between two points in time, including both psychological and physical components (Hill 1999). Selecting 'nurse sensitive' indicators seems key to choosing appropriate outcome measures (Wong et al. 2006) with some consensus regarding three main areas of clinical outcomes (Hill 1999, Urden 2001):

- Clinical outcomes (for example morbidity)
- Functional outcomes (for example activities of daily living)
- Cost and utilization (for example frequency of treatment/clinics)

However, suggestions for a fourth indicator vary between:

- Satisfaction outcomes (Hill 1999)
- Psychosocial outcomes (Urden 2001).

From this it seems that choosing the most appropriate clinical outcomes is crucial to assessing the effectiveness of nurse-led clinics and determining the potential value and possible differences between medical management. The first three indicators appear to be more traditional clinical outcome measures to compare medical (clinical) effectiveness and cost effectiveness of nurse-led versus medical services. However, the addition of a fourth indicator (satisfaction or psychosocial outcomes) may be the most important factor to show possible differences of quality or added value of nurse-led and medical clinics.

Evaluating nurse-led clinics

Despite the rapid increases in nurse-led clinics, there is little evidence of formal evaluation. The most common method of evaluation is to assess patient satisfaction through audits using a structured questionnaire that is created locally. However, establishing patient satisfaction in this way is highly likely to achieve positive results, therefore may convey little useful information regarding the effectiveness of the clinic, specific issues or areas for potential improvement.

Although clinical audits with structured questionnaires can be a useful way to evaluate nurse-led clinics, it is important to consider what outcomes should be assessed, and what questions are likely to elicit such information in a meaningful and unbiased way. Incorporating clinical and psychological outcomes will provide more meaningful data on the potential benefits of nurse-led clinics in relation to patients' experiences and clinical care, rather than solely focusing on patient satisfaction, however evaluating this is more challenging.

Faithfull and Hunt (2005) propose that nurse-led clinics may have a therapeutic value for patients where continuity, communication and trust in care are pivotal to dealing with uncertainly and the provision of therapeutic support, whilst others report how much patients value their relationship with the nurse (Wells et al. 2008, Cox et al. 2008). However, despite indications in the literature that some nurse-led clinics may improve patients' psychological distress (Cox et al. 2008), several studies show no differences in comparison to doctors (Helgessen et al. 2000; Brown et al. 2002; Baildam et al. 2004, Koinberg et al. 2004, Lewis et al. 2009, Beaver et al. 2009, Sheppard et al. 2009, Kimman et al. 2011). However, although there may be no difference in patients' psychological distress, nurses in one study are able to detect this more frequently than doctors (Baildam et al. 2004).

Determining the cost-effectiveness and resource utilisation within nurse-led clinics is also important, although this will require support from other health professionals and academics, such as health economists. There is a common perception that nurse-led clinics are a cheaper option than medical clinics due to differences in salary between the two professions, however evidence from randomised controlled trials shows no difference in the cost of doctor-led and nurse-led follow-up care (Moore et al. 2002, Baildam et al. 2004, Strand et al. 2011), since the difference in salary may be offset by other factors. When timings of consultations are given it seems that nurse-led clinics are deliberately set up to give patients at least twice as much time as medical clinics (Farrell 2014, Kimman et al. 2010, Palmer and Thain 2010, Beaver et al. 2009, Wells et al. 2008, Warren 2007, Coughlan 2005, Faithfull et al. 2001). In addition, some nurse-led clinics increased the use of resources such as blood tests (Strand et al. 2011) and other investigations, prescriptions or increased referrals to other health professionals (Campbell et al. 1999). Nevertheless, Faithfull et al. (2001) show a reduction of 31 per cent in the cost of nurse-led versus doctor-led care in radiotherapy clinics.

However, changing the mode of delivery with nurse-led clinics seems to be the greatest factor in influencing costs. Nurse-led telephone consultations for follow-up can be cost-effective (Cusack and Taylor 2010). Helgessen et al. (2000) identify a 37 percent reduction in costs in telephone consultations compared with face-to-face clinics.

The best way to evaluate nurse-led clinics is by undertaking academic nursing research, since research methods will enable the provision of data that is robust, credible and unbiased due to increased validity and reliability, particularly if the research is conducted by independent researchers. However this will require additional funding, research training and time to undertake, including data analysis, although will provide valuable evidence of nurse-led clinics. For example, incorporating qualitative research using interview and observational methods to evaluate nurse-led clinics has also shown disparities between what nurses think they do and what they actually do in practice (Farrell 2014).

Summary

Regulatory changes to professional practice together with key changes in legislation have provided the backdrop for developments in nursing practice, including nurse-led clinics. Nurses in the UK have been keen to embrace such developments and expand their current roles, or create new roles within advanced nursing practice. The timing of such developments also fitted well with reductions in junior doctors' hours to plug certain gaps in service provision, whilst providing additional opportunities for nurses. However it has not all been plain sailing since the majority of nurse-led clinics have been set up ad hoc with little planning, and based on doctor-nurse substitutions and medical models of care. There is no training for nurse-led clinics; therefore some nurses may struggle with some aspects, such as how to structure the consultation, changes in 'closed door' communication with patients, organisational aspects of nurse-led clinics and operational processes. One of the most important things to remember is that nurse-led clinics should not be set up in isolation, and although there may be only one nurse running the clinic it is teamwork that will keep it going.

References

Allinson V. (2004). Breast cancer: evaluation of a nurse-led family history clinic. *Journal of Clinical Nursing*. 13: 765–766.

Anderson B. (2010). The benefits to nurse-led telephone follow-up for prostate cancer. *British Journal of Nursing*. 19(17): 1085–1090.

Baildam A, Keeling F, Thompson L, Bundred N, Hopwood P. (2004). Nurse-led surgical follow-up clinics for women treated for breast cancer – a randomised controlled trial. *European Journal of Cancer*. 38 (Suppl. 3): S136–137.

Bala SV, Samuelson K, Hagell P, Svensson B, Fridlund B, Hesselgard K. (2012). The experience of care at nurse-led rheumatology clinics. *Musculoskeletal Care*. 10(4): 202–211.

Beaver K, Craven O, Witham G, Tomlinson M, Susnerwala S, Jones D, Luker K. (2007). Patient participation in decision making: views of health professionals caring for people with colorectal cancer. *Journal of Clinical Nursing*. 16(4): 725–733.

Beaver K, Tysver-Robinson D, Campbell M, Twomey M, Williamson S, Hindley A, Susnerwala S, Dunn G, Luker K. (2009). Comparing hospital and telephone follow up after treatment for breast cancer: randomised equivalence trial. *British Medical Journal*. 338: 3147–3156.

Belling R, McLaren S, Boudioni M, Woods L. (2012). Pan-London tuberculosis services: a service evaluation. *BMC Health Services Research*. 12: 203.

Booker J, Eardley A, Cowan R, Logue J, Wylie J, Caress AL. (2004). Telephone first post-intervention follow up for men who have had radical radiotherapy to the prostate: evaluation of a novel service delivery approach. *European Journal of Oncology Nursing*. 8(4): 325–333.

Brown L, Payne S, Royle G. (2002). Patient initiated follow up of breast cancer. *Psycho-Oncology*. 11: 346–355.

Campbell J, German L, Lane C. (1999). Radiotherapy outpatient review: a nurse-led clinic. *Nursing Standard*. 13(22): 39–44.

Challenor R, Henwood E, Burgess J, Clare D. (2006). Effective role redesign: an audit of outcomes following the introduction of a new nurse-led service. *International Journal of STD & AIDS*. 17(8): 555–557.

Chummun H. (2009). Hypertension – a contemporary approach to nursing care. *British Journal of Nursing*. 18(13): 784–789.

Clack G. (2009). Decision making in nursing practice: a case review. *Paediatric Nursing*. 21(5): 24–27.

Clark CE, Smith LF, Taylor RS, Campbell JL. (2011). Nurse-led interventions used to improve control of high blood pressure in people with diabetes: a systematic review and meta-analysis. *Diabetic Medicine*. 28(3): 250–261.

Corner J. (2003). The role of nurse-led care in cancer management. *Lancet Oncology*. 4(10): 631–636.

Coughlin C. (2005). Screening for familial cases of colorectal cancer: a new practice environment. *Cancer Nursing Practice*. 4(4): 35–39.

Courtney M, Carey N, Stenner K. (2009). Nurse prescriber-patient consultations: a case study in dermatology. *Journal of Advanced Nursing*. 65(6): 1207–1217.

Cox A, Bull E, Cockle-Hearne J, Knibb W, Potter C, Faithfull S. (2008). Nurse led telephone follow up in ovarian cancer: a psychosocial perspective. *European Journal of Oncology Nursing*. 12(5): 412–417.

Cox K, Wilson E, Heath L, Collier J, Jones L, Johnson I. (2006). Preferences for follow up after treatment for lung cancer: assessing the nurse-led option. *Cancer Nursing*. 29(3): 176–187.

Cusack M, Taylor C. (2010). A literature review of the potential of follow up in colorectal cancer. *Journal of Clinical Nursing*. 19(17–8): 2394–2405.

Department of Health. (2006). *Improving Patients' Access to Medicines: A Guide to Implementing Nurse and Pharmacist Independent Prescribing within the NHS in England*. London, DH.

Department of Health. (2007). *The Cancer Reform Strategy*. London, DH.

Department of Health. (2008). *High Quality Care for All: NHS Next Stage Review*. London, DH.

Department of Health. (2009). Impact Assessment of National Chemotherapy Advisory Group Recommendations. http//tinyurl.com/8a7pfyq [accessed 25.03.2012].

Duce K, Gouldstone A. (2006). A practical guide to carrying out skin-prick allergy testing. *Nursing Times*. 102(48): 28–29.

Edwall LL, Hellstrom AL, Ohrn I, Danielson E. (2008). The lived experience of the diabetes nurse specialist regular check-ups, as narrated by patients with type 2 diabetes. *Journal of Clinical Nursing*. 17(6): 772–781.

Faithfull S, Corner J, Meyer L, Huddart R, Dearnaley D. (2001). Evaluation of a nurse-led follow up for patients undergoing pelvic radiotherapy. *British Journal of Cancer*. 85(12): 1853–1864.

Faithfull S, Hunt G. (2005). Exploring nursing values in the development of a nurse-led service. *Nursing Ethics*. 12(5): 440–452.

Farrell C. (2014). *An exploration of oncology nurse specialists' roles in nurse-led chemotherapy clinics*. Unpublished PhD thesis, University of Manchester.

Farrell C, Lennan E. (2013). Nurse-led chemotherapy clinics: issues for the prescriber. *Nurse Prescribing*. 11(7): 561–566.

Ferguson A, Kearney N. (2000). Towards a European framework for cancer nursing. In *Cancer Nursing Practice: A Textbook for the Specialist Nurse*. (N. Kearney, A. Richardson, P. DiGiulio, eds), pp. 179–196. Edinburgh, Churchill Livingstone.

Griffith R, Tengnah C. (2013). District nurse clinics: accountability and practice. *British Journal of Community Nursing*. 18(2): 94–97.

Gulzar Z, Goff S, Njindou A, Hearty H, Rafi I, Savage R. Matta G, Ferras J, Hodgson S. (2007). Nurse-led cancer genetics clinics in primary and secondary care in varied ethnic population areas: interaction with primary care to improve ascertainment of individuals from ethnic minorities. *Familial Cancer*. 6(2): 205–212.

Hadjikoutis S, Smith PE. (2005). Approach to the patient with epilepsy in the outpatient department. *Postgraduate Medical Journal*. 81(957): 442–44.

Helgessen F, Andersson SO, Gustafsson O, Varenhorst E, Gobén B, Carnock S, Sehlstedt L, Carlsson P, Holmberg L, Johansson JE. (2000). Follow-up of prostate cancer patients by on-demand contacts with a specialist nurse: a randomized study. *Scandanavian Journal of Urology and Nephrology*. 34 (1): 55–61.

Hill M. (1999). Outcomes measurement requires nursing to shift to outcome-based practice. *Nursing Administration Quarterly*. 24: 1–16.

James ND, Guerro D, Brada M. (1994). Who should follow up cancer patients? Nurse specialist based outpatient care and the introduction of a phone clinic system. *Clinical Oncology*. 6: 283–287.

Jeyarajah S, Adams KJ, Higgins L, Ryan S, Leather AJ, Papagrigoriadis S. (2010). Prospective evaluation of a colorectal cancer nurse follow-up clinic. *Colorectal Disease*. 13(1): 31–38.

Kengne AP, Awah PK, Fezeu LL, Sobngwi E, Mbanya JC. (2009). Primary health care for hypertension by nurses in rural and urban sub-Saharan Africa. *Journal of Clinical Hypertension*. 11(10): 564–572.

Kimman ML, Bloebaum MM, Dirksen CD, Houben RM. (2010). Patient satisfaction with nurse-led telephone follow up after curative treatment for breast cancer. *BMC Cancer*. 10: 174.

Kimman ML, Dirksen CD, Voogd, C, Falger P, Gijsen BC, Thuring M, Lenssen A, van der Ent F, Verkeyn J, Haekens C, Hupperets P, Nuytinck JK, vanRiet Y, Brenninkmeijer SJ, Scheijmans LJ, Kessels A, Lambin P, Boersma LJ. (2011). Nurse-led telephone follow-up and an educational group programme after breast cancer treatment: results of a 2 x 2 randomised controlled trial. *European Journal of Cancer*. 47(7): 1027–1036.

Knowles G, Sherwood L, Dunlop MG, Dean G, Jodrell D, McLean C, Preston E. (2007). Developing and piloting a nurse-led model of follow-up in the multidisciplinary management of colorectal cancer. *European Journal of Oncology Nursing*. 11(3): 212–223.

Koelewijn-van Loon MS, van der Weijden T, van Steenkiste B, Ronda G, Winkens B, Severens JL, Wensing M, Elwyn G, Grol R. (2009). Involving patients in cardiovascular risk management with nurse-led clinics: a cluster randomized controlled trial. *Canadian Medical Association Journal*. 181(12): E267–274.

Koinberg IL, Fridlund B, Engholm GB, Holmberg L. (2004). Nurse-led follow up on demand or by a physician after breast cancer surgery: a randomised study. *European Journal of Oncology Nursing*. 8(2): 109–117; discussion 118–120.

Labhardt ND, Manga E, Ndam M, Balo JR, Bischoff A, Stoll B. (2009). Early assessment of the implementation of a national programme for the prevention of mother-to-child transmission of HIV in Cameroon and the effects of staff training: a survey in 70 rural health care facilities. *Tropical Medicine & International Health*. 14(3): 288–293.

Lane L, Minns S. (2010). Empowering advanced practitioners to set up nurse led clinics for improved outpatient care. *Nursing Times*. 106(13): 14–15.

Lewis R, Neal RD, Williams NH, France B, Wilkinson C, Hendry M, Russell D, Russell I, Hughes DA, Stuart NSA, Weller D. (2009). Nurse-led vs. conventional physician-ed follow up for patients with cancer: systematic review. *Journal of Advanced Nursing*. 65(4): 706–723.

MacLeod A, Branch A, Cassidy J, McDonald A, Mohammed N, MacDonald L. (2007). A nurse/pharmacy-led capecitabine clinic for colorectal cancer: results of a prospective audit and retrospective survey of patient experiences. *European Journal of Oncology Nursing*. 11: 247–254.

Mason JM, Freemantle N, Gibson JM. (2005). Specialist nurse-led clinics to improve control of hypertension and hyperlipidemia in diabetes: economic analysis of the SPLINT trial. *Diabetes Care*. 28(1): 40–46.

Moore S, Corner J, Fuller F. (1999). Development of nurse-led follow up in the management of patients with lung cancer. *Nursing Times Research*. 4: 432–444.

Moore S, Corner J, Haviland J, Wells M, Salmon E, Normand C, Brada M, O'Brien M, Smith I. (2002). *Nurse led follow up and conventional medical follow up in management of patients with lung cancer: randomised trial. BMJ*. 325(7373): 1145–1147.

Moore S, Wells M, Plant H, Fuller F, Wright M, Corner J. (2006). Nurse specialist led follow up in lung cancer: the experience of developing and delivering a new model of care. *European Journal of Oncology Nursing*. 10(5): 364–377.

Murchie P, Campbell NC, Ritchie LD, Thain J. (2005). Running nurse-led secondary prevention clinics for coronary heart disease in primary care: qualitative study of health professionals' perspectives. *British Journal of General Practice*. 55(516): 522–528.

National Chemotherapy Advisory Group (NCAG). (2009). *Chemotherapy services in England: Ensuring Quality and Safety. A Report from the National Chemotherapy Advisory Group*. London, Department of Health.

Ndosi M, Lewis M, Hale C, Quinn H, Ryan S, Emery P, Bird H, Hill J. (2011). A randomised, controlled study of outcome and cost effectiveness for RA patients attending nurse-led rheumatology clinics: study protocol of an ongoing nationwide multi-centre study. *International Journal of Nursing Studies*. 48(8): 995–1001.

Nursing and Midwifery Council. (2008). *The Code: Standards of Conduct, Performance and Ethics for Nurses and Midwives*. London, NMC.

O'Shea E, Coughlan M, Corrigan H, McKee G. (2012). Evaluation of a nurse-led haemophilia counselling service. *British Journal of Nursing*. 21(14): 864–866, 868–870.

Palmer C, Thain C. (2010). Strategies to ensure effective and empathetic delivery of bad news. *Cancer Nursing Practice*. 9(9): 24–27.

Raftery JP, Yao GL, Murchie P, Campbell NC, Ritchie LD. (2005). Cost effectiveness of nurse led secondary prevention clinics for coronary heart disease in primary care: follow up of a randomised controlled trial. *British Medical Journal*. 330(7493): 707.

Rogers J. (2008). The impact paediatric bowel care pathway. *Nursing Times*. 104(18): 46–47.

Sardell S, Sharpe G, Ashley S, Guerrero D, Brada M. (2000). Evaluation of a nurse-led telephone clinic in the follow up of patients with malignant glioma. *Clinical Oncology*. 12(1): 36–41.

Schadewaldt V, Schultz T. (2011). Nurse-led clinics as an effective service for cardiac patients: results from a systematic review. *International Journal of Evidence-Based Healthcare*. 9(3): 199–214.

Shakeel M, Newton JR, Clark D, Hussain A. (2008). Patients' satisfaction with the nurse-led aural care clinic. *Journal of Ayub Medical College*. 20(3): 81–83.

Sheppard C, Higgins B, Wise M, Yiangou C, Dubois D, Kilburn S. (2009). Breast cancer follow up: a randomised controlled trial comparing point of need access versus routine 6-monthly clinical review. *European Journal of Oncology Nursing*. 13: 2–8.

Shiu AT, Lee DT, Chau JP. (2012). Exploring the scope of expanding advanced nursing practice in nurse-led clinics: a multiple-case study. *Journal of Advanced Nursing*. 68(8): 1780–1792.

Stenner K, Courtenay M. (2008a). The role of inter-professionals relationships and support for nurse prescribing in acute and chronic pain. *Journal of Advanced Nursing*. 63(3): 276–283.

Stenner K, Courtenay M. (2008b). Benefits of nurse prescribing for patients in pain: nurses' views. *Journal of Advanced Nursing*. 63(1): 27–35.

Strand E, Nygren I, Bergkvist L, Smedh K. (2011). Nurse or surgeon follow up after rectal cancer: A randomized trial. *Colorectal Disease*. 13(9): 999–1003.

Tomlinson M, John Gibson G. (2006). Obstructive sleep apnoea syndrome: a nurse-led domiciliary service. *Journal of Advanced Nursing*. 55(3): 391–397.

Turner B, Wells P. (2012). Evaluating the efficacy of a telephone follow up clinic. *Cancer Nursing Practice*. 11(1): 32–35.

UKCC. (1992). *The Scope of Professional Practice*. UKCC, London.

Urden, L. (2001). Outcome evaluation: an essential component for CNS practice. *Clinical Nurse Specialist*. 15: 260–268.

Warren M. (2007). Breast cancer patient satisfaction with the nurse-led clinic for surgical histology. *Cancer Nursing Practice*. 6(7): 35–39.

Wells M, Donnan PT, Sharp L, Ackland C, Fletcher J, Dewar JA. (2008). A study to evaluate nurse-led on treatment review for patients undergoing radiotherapy for head and neck cancer. *Journal of Clinical Nursing*. 17(11): 1428–1439.

Williamson S, Twelvetree T, Thompson J, Beaver K. (2012). An ethnographic study exploring the role of ward-based advanced nurse practitioners in an acute medical setting. *Journal of Advanced Nursing*. 68(7): 1579–1588.

Winter H, Lavender V, Blesing C. (2011). Developing a nurse-led clinic for patients enrolled in clinical trials. *Cancer Nursing Practice*. 10(3): 20–24.

Wong FKY, Chung LCY. (2006). Establishing a definition for a nurse-led clinic: structure, process and outcome. *Nursing and Healthcare Management and Policy*. 358–369.

Woodward A, Wallymahmed M, Wilding JP, Gill GV. (2010). Nurse-led clinics for strict hypertension control are effective long term: a 7 year follow-up study. *Diabetic Medicine*. 27(8): 933–937.

Youngman S. (2004). The developing role of the renal diabetes nurse. *Edtna-Erca Journal*. 30(3): 169–172.

Chapter 8

The nature of nurse-led clinics in oncology

Carole Farrell

This chapter will be divided into different sections covering the core treatments in oncology, and also the development of nurse-led clinics to improve services for patients. This will be based on a review of the literature covering surgical, chemotherapy and radiotherapy nurse-led clinics, together with practical examples from clinical practice. There will also be additional sections on nurse-led follow-up clinics and nurse-led clinics for patients on clinical trials. However I would like to begin this chapter by sharing my own experience of developing and running several nurse-led clinics over the past ten years.

Developing and expanding nurse-led clinics at the Christie

I qualified as a nurse clinician in October 2003 and began to set up nurse-led clinics six months later. The developments happened in a step wise fashion, which relied on support from the medical consultant, changes to legislation, and practical opportunities . . . along with a great deal of hard work and determination on my part!

Developing protocol-led clinics

Whilst working within the medical clinics the consultant and I decided that patients on adjuvant chemotherapy didn't need to be seen in clinic at every cycle, therefore I set up a system where patients would be seen in clinic at the start, middle and end of chemotherapy, and they could be seen by chemotherapy nurses on other cycles. I created protocols for chemotherapy nurses, outlining their responsibilities regarding clinical management, including the clinical parameters for chemotherapy nurse-led care, and called this a 'protocol-led' clinic. The protocol-led clinic was used mainly for patients on adjuvant chemotherapy, since this was clinically the most straightforward. I had set up a separate clinic stream in the consultant's name for this so that we could clearly identify patients who did not need to be seen in clinic, but required chemotherapy and supportive medicines to be prescribed appropriately and in a timely manner. Having a separate list facilitated that, and the responsibility for future prescribing lay with the clinician who had last seen the patient in clinic. This was quite a radical step within the hospital at the time, and initially met with resistance from some nursing and medical colleagues, although protocol-led care is now well established and accepted within the hospital, and nationally.

Developing nurse-led chemotherapy clinics

As soon as we were allowed to have nurse-led clinics in our own name I saw this as a chance to streamline the medical clinics and set up my own nurse-led clinics. By this time the protocol-led clinics were established, running well and accepted by staff and patients. I wanted to take over responsibility for this and have my own nurse-led clinic running alongside it for adjuvant patients, which meant that I had the clinical responsibility for all patients on adjuvant chemotherapy within breast medical oncology. The time which I invested in fine-detail organisation and planning paid dividends, however I had to make some compromises initially to get it off the ground. The only room that was available in the outpatient department was under the stairs, although it did have a desk, chair and examination couch. I also had no help initially from the clinic nurses so I had to do everything myself, but it was a starting point. During the next 12 months my clinic was well established and accepted. I managed my own clinic list and the protocol-led list, enabling patients easy accessibility to see me if they had any problems and were on the protocol list.

Taking out all the adjuvant patients from the medical clinic into my nurse-led clinic had a huge impact on the medical clinics, reducing patient numbers allowed more time for individual consultations, reduced patients' waiting time and shaved hours off the finishing time of each clinic. In contrast my workload increased dramatically and I had to reduce some of my time spent in other medical clinics. I had also switched the clinic day/time to reduce pressure on the chemotherapy services, and set up another nurse-led chemotherapy clinic and protocol-led clinic on a different day to enable flexibility for patients and chemotherapy nurses with treatment days. The benefits for patients were clear due to reductions in waiting times, flexibility and continuity of care.

Developing nurse-led research clinics

During busy times and with one adjuvant clinical trial, I had support from the research nurses who would review some trial patients in clinic, which helped tremendously. Although they could not prescribe nor obtain informed consent, it demonstrated how skill mix can be used effectively in nurse-led clinics, and how different nursing roles can work together to improve patient care. This also demonstrated how nurse-led research clinics can work in practice by combining nurses' skills and roles.

Benefits of electronic prescribing in nurse-led clinics

I was also piloting electronic prescribing for the hospital, which meant that I could do most of the prescribing after the clinic. It also meant that I could check the day before clinic to see whether chemotherapy prescriptions had been completed, which reduced delays for patients.

Developing nurse-led radiotherapy clinics

Working across clinical and medical oncology also created benefits from nurse-led approaches. If patients in my clinic needed radiotherapy after chemotherapy I would discuss this with each patient before the end of their chemotherapy, provide written information and a plan to start radiotherapy four weeks after their final chemotherapy. Within the next week I would take the patients' notes and radiotherapy booking form to the clinical oncologist, provide a brief outline of the clinical history, and the booking form would be completed in a few minutes. I would also note on the form when the last cycle of chemotherapy is due and a provisional date to schedule the radiotherapy in order to avoid unnecessary delays. Although this created additional work for me it meant that patients would not need an additional appointment to see the radiotherapist during chemotherapy, thus saving time for both parties. It also improved continuity for patients since I covered everything with them in my clinic.

Developing nurse-led Herceptin (Trastuzumab) clinics

In 2006 I helped to establish nurse-led clinics for patients on adjuvant Trastuzumab, which was initially with one of the breast care nurses. Prior to our clinic the service was managed jointly between a pharmacist and the medical consultants, however there were some issues in relation to timely planning of cardiac assessments and clinical management. Meeting with all the breast oncologists I explained that to work effectively adjuvant Herceptin had to be totally nurse-led for the whole 12 months, outlining that the breast care nurse would see patients before starting Herceptin and the nurse clinician would undertake all clinical management during 12 months of treatment, after which the patient would be referred back to the consultant for follow-up care. I explained that patients would not be seen routinely in medical clinics during Herceptin, since patients would have regular clinical reviews/examination by the nurse clinician, and a protocol would be created to determine the structure of this service, frequency of cardiac assessments and criteria for suspending or stopping treatment and for referral to a cardiologist. All the oncologists agreed to this, which was no mean feat, and the nurse-led Herceptin clinics began.

The role of the breast care nurse was mainly information and support for all patients before starting Herceptin. This enabled consistency with information and access to the nurse-led service. The breast care nurse (BCN) would meet each patient during chemotherapy to explain about Herceptin, the nurse-led management and schedule of clinic appointments. The BCN would then liaise with the nurse clinician to arrange an echocardiogram and subsequently to prescribe Herceptin if the echocardiogram was normal. The BCN would liaise with the patient and schedulers to start cycle one.

The nurse clinician was responsible for managing patients during Herceptin. Initially echocardiograms and nurse-led clinic appointments were every three months, however these have become less frequent over time with later advances (see chapter 9). All Herceptin prescribing was completed by the nurse clinician, and all echocardiograms requested, results reviewed and treatment authorised. Patients attending the nurse-led clinics had a clinical examination, including respiratory and cardiovascular if necessary. I would inform patients of the echocardiogram results, explore, discuss and manage any side effects or symptoms, and explore and address any psychosocial concerns or other issues. If patients were also on endocrine treatment I would discuss this with them, exploring and discussing any concerns regarding possible side effects or other issues. In managing the patient's treatment I was also responsible for suspending or stopping Herceptin if there was a significant drop in the patient's left ventricular ejection fraction. After explaining this to the patient and outlining the plan to address this, I would inform the consultant and refer the patient to a cardiologist if necessary. More recently, in accordance with local and national guidelines, I would usually prescribe an angiotensin converting enzyme (ACE) inhibitor for the patient, and liaise with the patients' general practitioner for dose titration and further monitoring.

Development of nurse-led follow-up clinics

I started a separate nurse-led clinic for patients who needed routine follow-up after completion of chemotherapy and those who had completed Herceptin. This ensured continuity of care from starting chemotherapy until discharge from breast medical oncology. However, at the end of chemotherapy I offered patients a choice of continuing nurse-led care or returning to the medical clinics, since I wanted to take into account patients' preferences. Only one patient expressed a wish to transfer to the medical clinic, which illustrates the value of continuity.

The continuity of chemotherapy and follow-up clinics enabled me to have a greater understanding of patients' experiences and recovery after treatment. It facilitated greater discussion of the chronic side-effects of treatment such as fatigue, peripheral neuropathy, arthralgia, and other issues, such as menopausal symptoms, returning to work, caring for children or elderly parents, and psychological issues such as relationships, psychological distress, coping and uncertainty about the future.

For patients who were on adjuvant endocrine treatment the continuity facilitated symptom monitoring and management, which in some cases resulted in suspending or stopping endocrine treatment, or switching to another drug if appropriate. In such cases I would usually monitor patients' symptoms through telephone consultations until another clinic appointment was required. This provided greater flexibility and convenience for patients. I also realised that continuity of care increased patients' trust and confidence; therefore they were more likely to contact me if they had any worries or concerns. In some cases this was managed by a telephone consultation, however if patients needed, or wanted, to be seen in person I could fit them in one of my clinics.

If I suspected possible recurrence of the patient's cancer I would discuss my concerns with the patient, arrange appropriate investigations and explore their feelings and concerns. Once I had the results I would phone the patient with an appointment for my clinic to discuss the results; if the results indicate cancer recurrence I would discuss the implications and possible treatment with the patient, arrange full staging with other investigations, then discuss with the consultant and transfer the patient back to the medical clinic.

However the majority of adjuvant patients continued in my follow-up clinics for several years until it was time to discharge them from medical oncology and transfer back to the surgeons for ongoing care.

Although my nurse-led clinics were very successful I did not undertake any rigorous evaluation, which means I have no published evidence to demonstrate this. I embarked on a PhD thinking that I could evaluate my clinics within the course, thus achieving two aims concurrently, however this was foolish. After starting the PhD I was advised to focus on other nurses and nurse-led clinics, rather than my own clinical practice, therefore I had no time to evaluate my own clinical work. Nevertheless I do have evidence of nurse-led clinics nationally from the results of a survey of oncology specialist nurses who were running nurse-led clinics, and results from an ethnographic study of nurse-led chemotherapy clinics in the UK (Farrell 2014).

Survey of nurse-led oncology clinics

A survey of 79 oncology specialist nurses in the UK who conducted nurse-led clinics show the majority of clinics were for routine follow-up (see Figure 8.1).

Section 1: Chemotherapy nurse-led clinics

This section will begin with a brief summary explaining the basic elements of chemotherapy treatment, implications for clinical practice and impact of government policies. Underpinned by current evidence from the author's PhD research, this section will provide a comprehensive review of nurse-led chemotherapy clinics, clarifying the nature of nurse-led chemotherapy. This will include extracts from nurses who have established their own chemotherapy nurse-led clinics, highlighting different models of care and recommendations for clinical practice.

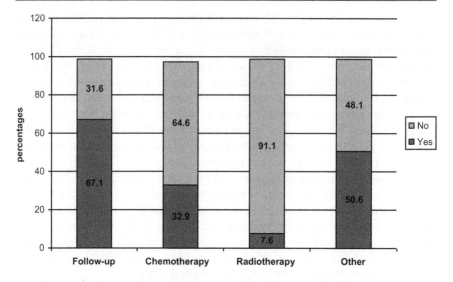

Figure 8.1 The nature of nurse-led clinics

Source: (adapted from Farrell 2014)

Systemic anti-cancer treatment (SACT)

Chemotherapy has traditionally been one of the main treatments in oncology alongside surgery and radiotherapy. Patients will have a course of chemotherapy where each treatment is referred to as a cycle and several cycles make up a course of treatment (NCEPOD 2008). The different types of chemotherapy drugs used for s course of treatment is known as the chemotherapy regimen, and the frequency of each cycle of chemotherapy can range from once a week to once every three or four weeks, although there are other standard variations in frequency. The number of cycles for each chemotherapy regimen is determined by evidence from clinical trials, and there are numerous chemotherapy drugs and different schedules and regimens for each cancer group. Chemotherapy drugs may be given alone or in combination, and with curative or palliative intent. In potentially curative treatment maximum tolerated doses are used to achieve greater efficacy, however this carries a greater risk of morbidity and mortality from treatment (NCEPOD 2008). In contrast, palliative chemotherapy aims to relieve or delay the onset of symptoms, therefore drug doses are often reduced to minimise treatment-related toxicities (NCEPOD 2008).

The side-effects of chemotherapy vary according to each regimen; however they can also vary in severity, with individual differences for each patient (NCEPOD 2008). The common side-effects include fatigue, hair loss, nausea and vomiting, mouth ulceration, diarrhoea and bone marrow suppression. An international grading system by the National Cancer Institute (NCI) in the United States has provided a standard grading scale to assess toxicities (NCI 2009), which provides consistency amongst health professionals in recording chemotherapy-related toxicities, and can facilitate decisions to defer, stop or dose reduce chemotherapy. In addition, systemic treatments now include a variety of intravenous biological agents, or targeted therapies, which have implications for chemotherapy nurses and clinical services (Vickers et al. 2012).

A study by the National Confidential Enquiry into Patient Outcome and Death (NCEPOD) in 2008 reviewed the care of patients who died within 30 days of receiving SACT. The report highlighted safety issues, including 43 per cent (220/514) of patients who had grade three or four treatment-related toxicity, and 36 per cent (97/267) of cases where toxicities had not been recorded (NCEPOD 2008). Alongside this, a report by the National Chemotherapy Advisory Group (2009) highlighted issues within chemotherapy services, making 20 recommendations to improve quality and safety. Some of the recommendations included prescribing chemotherapy where chemotherapy regimens require approval by cancer networks and prescribers must follow clear guidelines (DH 2009, 2003). NCEPOD (2008) also recommends that junior medical staff should not be authorised to initiate SACT, although there are no clear recommendations for nurses.

Policy implications for nurse-led chemotherapy services

Endorsement of nurse-led chemotherapy by the National Chemotherapy Advisory Group (NCAG 2009) was an important landmark for oncology nursing, although it represents significant challenges for nurses to deliver quality and safety improvements recommended by NCAG. Approximately 4,000 staff in 200 hospitals in the UK are involved in administering chemotherapy, which is a major responsibility within the NHS (Lennan and McPhelim 2012). However, a lack of consistency in systems to categorize and commission chemotherapy service delivery has created variability in the organisation of chemotherapy services in the UK (Lennan and McPhelim 2012).

Developments in nurse-led chemotherapy services have arisen ad hoc and have been poorly evaluated; therefore it is difficult to appreciate their clinical impact and effectiveness. Furthermore the term 'nurse-led' is open to interpretation, with great disparities in scope of clinical practice, autonomy and responsibilities, which is creating confusion. Whilst some nurses appear to have fully autonomous nurse-led chemotherapy services, other nurses may not be able to prescribe independently, therefore may rely more on support from medical staff.

In the UK the administration of chemotherapy is usually undertaken by nurses (Wiseman et al. 2005), however the clinical management of patients undergoing chemotherapy is mainly undertaken by doctors. In recent years some of this responsibility has been devolved to senior nurses who may prescribe chemotherapy and supportive medication, assess toxicities of treatment and other aspects of clinical management through 'nurse-led' clinics (Lennan et al. 2012). The Cancer Reform Strategy (DH 2007) recognises the potential variability in current chemotherapy services and recommends the development of a 'strategic framework' for chemotherapy service delivery. Given the current developments in cancer nursing, it seems important that nurse-led chemotherapy services are taken into account within national strategic planning and commissioning processes. This seems to have particular merit given the emphasis placed on continuity of care by specialist nurses and the importance of patients' knowledge of, and access to, psychosocial and financial support.

Fitzsimmons et al. (2005) reported mixed opinions from patients regarding the concept of nurse-led chemotherapy clinics within a feasibility study of nurse-led chemotherapy clinics. However, this may reflect a lack of understanding of nurses' roles since patients regarded nurses as different but complementary to doctors.

The variability in chemotherapy provision in the UK presents an increasing challenge in view of limitations in capacity and resources at cancer centres and units, which leads to greater consideration for nurse-led models of care in relation to chemotherapy administration and clinical management of patients in outpatient departments. Although this creates a great potential for nurses to develop their practice and set up nurse-led clinics, it is important to ensure that adequate training, preparation and support for such posts are provided to keep pace with professional and clinical developments.

Aims of nurse-led chemotherapy clinics

The aim of nurse-led chemotherapy clinics is to assess patients during chemotherapy, ascertain treatment-related toxicities and determine whether patients are fit to continue with the chemotherapy treatment. From my research, the main reason given for setting up nurse-led chemotherapy clinics was to alleviate problems in the medical clinics, which appeared to stem from a reduction in medical staff and increasing clinical demands and resulted in many clinics exceeding capacity. However there were differences in how nurse-led chemotherapy clinics were set up, which may explain differences in consultations with patients.

Research on nurse-led chemotherapy clinics

Given the lack of research on nurse-led chemotherapy clinics and variability in clinical practice locally and nationally, I conducted an ethnographic study using four geographical locations in the UK (Farrell 2014). Incorporating interviews with nurses and observations of their nurse-led chemotherapy clinics provided objective evidence of the nature of nurses' roles and operational aspects of nurse-led clinics. This revealed some differences in perceptions between interview reports and observations of clinical practice, particularly in relation to communication skills. For example several nurses perceived that they provided holistic assessments and care, but there was no evidence of this during observations (Farrell 2014). Similarly there were examples of poor communication skills, including blocking, of which nurses seemed unaware, which contrasted with their own perceptions of good communication skills.

Nurse-patient consultations

In one location the nurse-led clinic focused primarily on the administration of chemotherapy in an open ward area, however nurses 'reviewed' patients immediately prior to chemotherapy administration. Although there were curtains between the beds they were not used; there was a lack of privacy for individual consultations between nurses and patients, with little space between the beds, and nurses often sat on the patient's bed during their consultation. Consultations with patients were brief and focused on chemotherapy side-effects, which were assessed in a structured checklist, which often blocked communication.

In contrast, other locations had separate nurse-led review consultations, which were all conducted in a private room within the chemotherapy unit or in the outpatient department. This setting was similar to medical clinics, where each clinic room had an examination couch, desk with a computer and small chairs for the patient and relatives. This setting offered privacy during consultations between nurses and patients/relatives, and nurses referred to this as a 'closed door consultation,' where patients were given an appointment to attend the nurse-led clinic. This type of setting led to a different type of consultation with patients and reflected a medical consultation. Although patients would have their bloods taken and checked by the nurse prior to chemotherapy, the chemotherapy administration would be undertaken later that day or on a different day.

There were also significant differences between the number of consultations per nurse and the average time for nurse-patient consultations, which ranged from three minutes to one hour. In some cases this duration of consultations was influenced by the number of patients in the clinic (Farrell 2014) (see Table 8.1).

This shows the number of consultations per nurse at each location. Consultation times for each nurse indicate the range, mean and total time taken, which does not include time between consultations. Several nurses perceived that their nurse-led chemotherapy clinics provided patients with more time to talk. Observations showed that the majority of nurses' clinics were small and appointment slots were longer than medical clinics. However, in some cases the nurse-led clinics only had one or two patients and nurses expressed concerns regarding the viability of their clinics:

'We don't see enough patients and they [consultants] don't see that we're doing enough to alleviate . . . I think they see it more as a reduction in their

Table 8.1 Nurse-patient consultations observed at each location

Location	Number of nurses	Consultations observed	Time: range (minutes)	Time: mean (minutes)
1	3	39	3.04–56.00	17.36
2	4	7	10.32–39.18	24.23
3	3	12	8.42–60.43	22.94
4	2	3	8.32–26.14	16.50
TOTAL	**12**	**61**	**3.04–60.43**	**20.26**

workload so . . . 'cause if we're not seeing enough patients then for them that's not an effective clinic.' [I.L4.N13]

Some nurses perceived that the selection of patients for nurse-led clinics was the key to success, together with careful consideration of clinic numbers. To build their confidence nurses often started off with small numbers and specific patient criteria. Protocols were created so that patients could be carefully selected from one chemotherapy regimen, which would also reduce the number of potential patients.

'I think it started with the adjuvant patients first. They've got no disease present . . . you're basically steering them through a course of chemotherapy, monitoring the toxicities and managing the side-effects' [I.L2.N4]

'We felt that adjuvant patients was the right way to go because we assumed that they would have less disease-related toxicities than metastatic patients' [I.L4.N12]

Once the clinic was established, the aim was to increase the number of patients and expand the referral criteria to incorporate more complex regimens, and patients. However, some of the nurse-led clinics continued with small numbers due to a low volume of referrals from medical clinics.

'Today there is only one patient but we have days when we have five, six patients which is fine, that's manageable between two of us' [I.L4.N15]

'There's still problems recruiting patients, and I think that's because the group of patients we see is quite narrow' [I.L4.N13]

(Farrell 2014, p234)

Small numbers within nurse-led clinics will raise questions regarding the cost-effectiveness, resource utilisation and sustainability. However, gaining an appropriate number of patients for each nurse-led clinic is challenging. If numbers are too low nurses could face criticism, yet if there are too many patients nurse-led clinics will run late and increase waiting time for patients. In addition, increasing demand from medical colleagues can also be challenging if patients are too complex for nurses to manage effectively and safely. Therefore it seems a fine balance to maintain an appropriate number of patients to match the skill mix within each nurse-led clinic.

In some locations there was evidence of the need to assess nurses' competency within nurse-led clinics, which was either undertaken by a medical consultant or chemotherapy nurse manager. However there is no national standardisation regarding this and regional/national variations are evident.

Protocols and documentation

Nurses at three locations worked to a written protocol for their nurse-led clinics, although there were individual differences in protocols from each location.

The local protocols were established to determine the type of patients doctors would refer to nurse-led clinics, and protocols included specific guidelines for nurses' clinical management during chemotherapy, such as parameters for blood results and chemotherapy toxicities. This enabled nurses to work independently within these guidelines and refer back to the doctors if anything arose outside of them, such as unexpected events / toxicities or suspected progressive disease.

However, there were no protocols for nurse-led clinics at one location where nurses undertook the whole patient management for all patients receiving chemotherapy within one cancer group, since nurses considered their autonomy and level of clinical responsibilities to be on a par with medical colleagues, therefore had high levels of clinical decision-making.

The documentation to assess patients within nurse-led clinics was similar to documentation by medical staff in relation to assessing the patient's physical performance status and chemotherapy toxicities, which was recorded in the patients' notes or electronic patient records. Some hospitals had electronic records which included chemotherapy toxicities; therefore nurses completed these for each patient following the consultation (Farrell 2014).

Informed consent and prescribing in chemotherapy clinics

The main forms of consent are verbal and written. However tacit consent is interpreted as implied cooperation, for example a patient holding out his/her arm whilst the nurse takes a blood sample. Written consent is required when the treatment or care involves potential risks for the patient or if it is complex. Similarly, written informed consent is a requirement for patients who participate in clinical trials or research studies. In all cases, the written consent stands as a record that discussions have taken place, including documentation of the patient's choice (NMC 2015). However if a person refuses treatment a written record of this must be documented in the patient's notes, including discussions held and decisions made.

Informed consent should be regarded as a process rather than a single event, and patients should have sufficient time to consider information given about treatments, such as chemotherapy, and have the opportunity to ask questions before giving their consent (NMC 2015). Nurses may have various levels of involvement in the informed consent process, depending on their role and clinical responsibilities. The majority of nurses will be involved in providing information and checking patients' understanding during consent processes, irrespective of whether tacit, verbal or written consent is required. However obtaining written informed consent from patients requires training and approvals at hospital Trust level, and should include a process of ongoing monitoring, although operational policies are likely to vary nationally and internationally. For example, our Trust requires nurses to undergo training led by a designated senior nurse or medical consultant; a designated medical consultant provides written approval of the nurse's competence to consent to specific procedures and/or treatments, with ongoing annual appraisals and written updates documenting nurses' competence.

My research on nurse-led chemotherapy clinics identified similar differences regarding the process of obtaining informed consent. At one location doctors had responsibility for consenting patients whilst at another this was the sole responsibility of nurses running the clinic. However, there was also variability in the other locations; sometimes this was undertaken by the nurse and other times by the doctors, although nurses sometimes had to check whether it had been completed.

Prescribing practices varied across all four locations; at one location nurses could prescribe freely provided it was within their area of competence, whilst nurses at two locations were not allowed to prescribe the first cycle of chemotherapy, although they could prescribe other cycles of chemotherapy. However, at one location nurse prescribing was severely restricted by medical consultants, which meant that they could only prescribe from a limited hospital formulary designated for nurse prescribers and determined by medical consultants:

> 'We have to stick to our own protocols, our own personal P Formulary . . . [if] we want to add more onto our P Formulary we have to apply to do . . . it's very very frustrating because the process is so slow and I think it's holding us back if you consider the amount of training that the nurses have gone through'
>
> [I.L2.N4, p252]

These restrictions caused frustration and also made nurses more dependent on doctors. In some cases it created additional waiting for patients, for example if nurses wanted to amend a patient's antiemetics and this drug was not on their permitted formulary, they had to find a doctor to prescribe it.

However the implications of being unable to prescribe independently are illustrated by the following quotation:

> 'I don't prescribe . . . so I do the assessment toxicity scale and then I ask the doctor to prescribe it'
>
> [I.L4.N14, p252]

This nurse had not completed the prescribing course, therefore had to ask colleagues to prescribe chemotherapy and any supportive medication that the patient may need, which caused delays for those patients (Farrell 2014).

Different levels of nurse-led chemotherapy clinics

The findings from observations and interviews with nurse participants suggest that there are four different levels of nurse-led chemotherapy clinics, which represent four levels from novice to expert depending on nurses' skills, clinical responsibilities and level of autonomy (Farrell 2014) (see Figure 8.2). It was also clearly evident from this research that with increasing medicalization of nurses' roles we lose the essence of nursing, therefore it is crucial that nurses' strive to maintain the fundamental nursing values and philosophy of nursing when expanding their roles and developing nurse-led clinics.

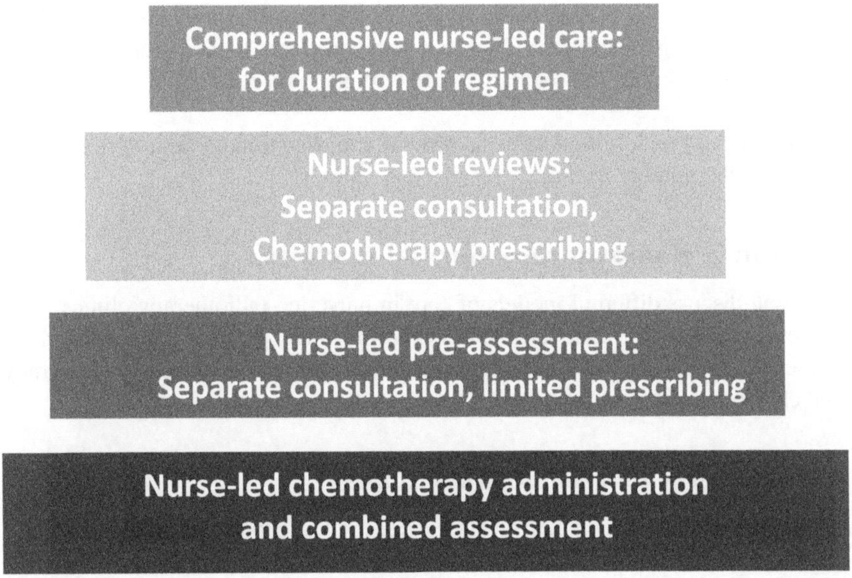

Comprehensive nurse-led care:
for duration of regimen

Nurse-led reviews:
Separate consultation,
Chemotherapy prescribing

Nurse-led pre-assessment:
Separate consultation, limited prescribing

Nurse-led chemotherapy administration
and combined assessment

Figure 8.2 Four levels of nurse-led chemotherapy clinics

Level 1 Nurse-led chemotherapy administration. No separate appointments to see patients for assessment review. Follows a checklist to assess symptoms. Follows a structured protocol for criteria to go ahead with chemotherapy.

Level 2 Nurse-led pre-assessment undertaken as a separate consultation with patients. Follows a checklist to assess symptoms. Follows a structured protocol for criteria to go ahead with chemotherapy. However, nurses need to check with medical staff if chemotherapy needs to be deferred or dose amended. Nurses unable to prescribe chemotherapy independently, and unable to undertake clinical examinations.

Level 3 Nurse-led chemotherapy reviews prior to chemotherapy. This is a separate consultation to assess symptoms and elicit patients' concerns. Nurses do not use a structured checklist, ask more open questions and make decisions whether to go ahead with chemotherapy or defer treatment, according to the protocol. In addition they can undertake informed consent for chemotherapy. However nurses cannot independently stop chemotherapy or amend treatment doses without discussion with medical staff. Nurses can prescribe and are trained in clinical examination skills so they can manage an episode of care, although the patient is still under the care of a medical consultant.

Level 4 Totally nurse-led chemotherapy clinics. Nurses are completely independent and responsible for patients during the whole of their chemotherapy regimen. Can undertake comprehensive assessments of patients, take informed consent, and utilise a higher level of decision-making in that they can stop, defer or amend the dose of chemotherapy without speaking to a doctor. They can admit patients without further medical consultation, and regularly liaise with the patient's GP.

This method of levelling aims to provide a basic structure and definition for nurse-led chemotherapy clinics.

Section 2: Radiotherapy nurse-led clinics

This will discuss different models of care in nurse-led radiotherapy clinics, with evidence from the literature and examples from clinical practice. This will include a brief outline of nurse-led clinics for patients receiving concurrent radiotherapy and chemotherapy treatments.

Nurses' roles within radiotherapy clinics

Whilst there is some information on nurses' roles and autonomy within nurse-led radiotherapy clinics, information on nurses' interactions and communication with patients is limited. This is due to limited evidence in the literature and the design of published studies, including how the findings are reported. Although Faithfull and Hunt (2005) go some way to addressing this when identifying professional values integral to nurse-led care, there are still gaps in the fine details of nurse-led interactions which would provide a greater understanding of nurses' roles within nurse-led clinics.

From the literature the role of the nurse seems to vary in each of the studies reviewed, often depending on how much autonomy nurses have within their clinic. Greater autonomy is evident where nurses take on more responsibility for patients' treatment (Faithfull et al. 2001; Faithfull and Hunt 2005; Wells et al. 2008), or conduct a specific nurse-led programme over several weeks (Lee et al. 2011; Seibeck and Peterson 2009).

The therapeutic value of nurse-led interactions is identified in two studies of patients undergoing radiotherapy (Faithfull and Hunt 2005; Sharp and Tishelman 2005), although this seems a difficult concept to define and suggests that further consideration is needed in relation to meeting patients' needs. Koinberg et al. (2002) identifies that patients' needs include trust, security and reassurance in addition to support, which fits with patients' desire for continuity since regular contact with a nurse should facilitate the development of trust, support and reassurance. One of the main advantages of nurses managing patients' treatment is the continuity of care, which enhances the nurse-patient relationship (Faithfull and Hunt 2005; Wells et al. 2008; Earnshaw and Stephenson 1997; Egan and Dowling 2005; Faithfull et al. 2001).

Radiotherapy nurse-led clinics: practical implications

There are three stages that nurses may be involved in the clinical management of radiotherapy: pre-treatment, during radiotherapy treatment and post-treatment.

However there is limited research evidence on nurses' roles within radiotherapy. I have divided this into three for the purpose of discussing how nurses' roles and responsibilities may vary in relation to nurse-led management; however there may be continuity of nurse-led care across the three stages.

Pre-radiotherapy treatment

Prior to staring radiotherapy patients must be aware of what the treatment will be, including how and when it is given, the duration of each treatment, what side-effects are likely to happen, when they usually occur, the possible severity of side-effects and how they will be managed. Specialist nurses can play an important part with this by tailoring information to each patient's needs to increase their understanding, providing written information and contact numbers for future contact if required. However, in some centres contact with specialist nurses pre-radiotherapy is ad hoc and patients rely on medical staff for their information needs.

To date there is no evidence of nurse-led radiotherapy clinics prior to treatment, and no comparison with medical clinics, therefore we can only speculate about the potential benefits of nurse-led clinics and use anecdotal examples from clinical practice.

Specialist nurse role

As a breast cancer clinical nurse specialist part of my clinical practice would be to discuss radiotherapy treatment with patients when they attended breast oncology clinics. Patients would be referred to a radiotherapy oncologist for a course of radiotherapy following breast surgery. In some cases this was immediately after surgery, however if patients required chemotherapy the radiotherapy would be given following this. Patients under the care of a medical oncologist would be given a separate clinic appointment with a clinical oncologist (radiotherapist) to plan the radiotherapy treatment, which was often during their chemotherapy. As a specialist nurse I would see patients with the oncologist, act as a chaperone during breast examination and discuss the radiotherapy treatment in more detail after the oncologists' consultation. Patients would then have a written information booklet and my contact number, and I would ask patients to contact me if needed during or following the radiotherapy. However, given the high number of patients with breast cancer at the hospital trust (approximately 2,000 new patients each year) it was impossible to see everyone, which created concerns about equity of access. This may not be an issue in smaller cancer units.

Advanced nurse practitioner role

As a nurse clinician (ANP) I had greater responsibilities in relation to patients undergoing radiotherapy. I would see new patients referred for radiotherapy after breast surgery when I worked within clinical oncology, however I would do a clinical examination and help to complete the radiotherapy booking form in addition to providing verbal and written information, and exploring patients' concerns. In those clinics I had similar medical responsibilities, and saw the same type of patients, as medical colleagues; however my consultations were often longer since I spent more time explaining and discussing information with patients and exploring their concerns. Although I covered some of the specialist nurses' (CNS) role and responsibilities during my consultations, I worked very closely with the CNSs in clinic. Sometimes the CNS would come into the consultation with me and other times I would tell her about the patient and discuss any issues. Due to the nature of nurses' roles the boundaries will be blurred between CNS and ANPs, which requires careful negotiation and sensitivity to avoid any misunderstanding or duplication of clinical tasks and practice.

I think the greatest impact of my ANP role in relation to patients requiring radiotherapy came from working between clinical and medical oncology and developing my nurse-led chemotherapy clinics. I developed a 'fast track' system for patients pre-radiotherapy, where I would provide written and verbal information at an appropriate point during chemotherapy, and within an existing appointment in my nurse-led clinic, and then complete the radiotherapy booking form with the consultant at a mutually convenient time. This enabled me to improve patients' experiences by reducing waiting times and the number of clinic visits, improving the timing of radiotherapy planning and treatment post chemotherapy, providing greater continuity for patients and reducing the throughput in the clinical oncology clinic. Although this greatly increased my workload, the benefits for patients, colleagues and service delivery were worthwhile.

During radiotherapy treatment

Symptom management is a considerable part of nurse-led clinics in radiotherapy, although there may be variability in the clinic's remit. During radiotherapy patients are reviewed weekly to determine how they are tolerating the treatment and assess side-effects. However, the introduction of nurse-led clinics allows nurses to be more flexible with appointments, which increases interventions (Campbell et al. 1999), allows the addition of telephone monitoring (Faithfull et al. 2001; Faithfull and Hunt 2005) and facilitates longer and more frequent consultations (Wells et al. 2008). However, although greater continuity of care was evident in nurse-led clinics, there was no difference in patients' quality of life (Faithfull et al. 2001). In addition, whilst some studies show high levels of patient satisfaction and acceptability with nurse-led clinics, there are no comparisons with traditional medical clinics (Egan and Dowling 2005).

Providing more time for patients facilitates greater information exchange within nurse-led clinics (Faithfull et al. 2001) and enable increased communication of information to GPs (Wells et al. 2008). Although there appear to be no significant differences in psychological well-being or quality of life within nurse-led radiotherapy clinics, patients seem to value their relationship with the nurse (Wells et al. 2008), and there is evidence of therapeutic support (Faithfull and Hunt 2005).

During radiotherapy, studies show that patients liked the openness of nurse-led clinics and found it easy to talk to the nurse (Fletcher and Hornsby 2007, Campbell et al. 1999). The way that nurse-led clinics are set up may increase accessibility, and the addition of telephone surveillance can also facilitate this (Faithfull et al. 2001). Continuity for patients may be greater within nurse-led clinics, which may not be possible within medical clinics.

Evidence from the literature demonstrates that nurses can work in different ways in the clinical management of patients during radiotherapy treatment, and there are examples of different nurse-led models of care (Faithfull et al. 2001, Wells et al. 2008, Fletcher and Hornsby 2007). The structure of radiotherapy treatment requires regular monitoring of patients to assess toxicities and ensure appropriate symptom management. Traditionally these were usually quick appointments with a doctor and focused on skin reactions and the physical effects of treatment. In addition, contact with specialist nurses was ad hoc and infrequent.

With the development of nurses', and allied health professionals', roles, this has led to nurse-led innovations in the care of patients during radiotherapy. In some cancer centres ANPs or therapy radiographers will undertake clinical reviews during radiotherapy instead of a doctor (Fletcher and Hornsby 2007). The frequency of reviews will vary according to each individual; once a week is usually the minimum frequency during the course of radiotherapy, however patients may be seen more frequently depending on the severity of side-effects, symptoms and patients' needs. The ability and availability of designated ANPs or allied health professionals (AHPs) to see patients ad hoc in addition to planned appointments will ensure prompt assessment and symptom management, thus reducing unnecessary waiting time for patients. In addition the continuity of care is improved since patients are more likely to see the same person each week, which should improve patients' trust and confidence, which may provide greater reassurance for patients.

The severity of radiotherapy toxicities will be influenced by the site of cancer, type of radiotherapy and treatment site, in addition to the individual reaction and sensitivity experienced by each patient. Symptom management is more effective when symptoms are identified early and treatment given promptly. Nurse-led involvement can play a crucial role in facilitating appropriate symptom management, for example pain, fatigue, gastrointestinal problems such as diarrhoea, nutritional problems, difficulty swallowing or eating. Similarly, nurse-led care can promote discussions about skin care and managing skin reactions, including topical treatments and dressings. In such situations non-medical prescribing is useful to reduce waiting time for patients and streamline clinical service delivery.

In addition to physical assessments and symptom management, nurse-led reviews offer greater opportunities for person-centred compassionate care, particularly regarding psychological, social and financial issues and concerns. However, this will depend on nurses' communication skills in picking up patients' cues and identifying/exploring their concerns. A nurse-led service in radiotherapy can also offer a combination of face-to-face clinics and telephone monitoring, which may be particularly useful when patients are struggling with side-effects.

There is an increase in the number of patients undergoing radiotherapy concurrently with chemotherapy, which may present additional challenges, for example in patients with head and neck cancers. Due to the complexity of treatment a multidisciplinary approach is required; however nurse-led clinics can be including in the management plan, for example where a nurse clinician (ANP) manages the patients' course of chemotherapy (Farrell 2014).

Post-radiotherapy treatment

One of the greatest challenges for patients undergoing radiotherapy is that the peak of the radiotherapy effects comes at the end of treatment and continues for several weeks later. During my work as a specialist nurse and nurse clinician, this created concerns for numerous patients and seemed to be one of the most frequent reasons for patients to phone specialist nurses for advice. Nurse-led telephone consultations may go some way to addressing issues in the first few weeks after radiotherapy, however nurses rely on patients to provide accurate reports of their symptoms, including self-assessment of their skin. In the majority of cases there is likely to be no problem with this, however wherever possible it is better to see patients face-to-face in order to assess their skin and document the findings in the patient's notes. This will also provide an opportunity to identify and explore patients' concerns, which again is easier to do, and more accurate, face-to-face than by telephone.

Some specialist nurses do not undertake any proactive telephone monitoring of patients during, and post, radiotherapy, which places the onus on patients to phone if they experience any problems. Patients who phone specialist nurses are highly likely to receive appropriate advice and symptom management, however there are still many patients who fail to contact health professionals and struggle on their own. There are many reasons for this, including patients who perceive that this is a normal reaction to the treatment, and that nothing can be done, therefore there is no point telephoning someone; some patients perceive specialist nurses to be busy with other patients who may need their help more, therefore they do not wish to be a burden; some patients may prefer their own privacy to cope on their own, and other patients may not want to leave a message on the nurses' voicemail if the phone is not answered immediately. One method of addressing this is nurse-led proactive telephone monitoring in the first few weeks after completion of radiotherapy. If this is undertaken in a structured way it can be incorporated into nurses' routine clinical practice (Booker et al. 2004; Faithfull et al. 2001) to provide a convenient, controlled and planned environment for clinical management. Being proactive rather than reactive may also reduce the number of urgent ad hoc telephone calls and crisis interventions. However, it is important that the potential benefits of such innovations are recognised and commissioned, therefore potential cost-savings and direct patient benefits are key to this process.

Section 3: Surgical nurse-led clinics

This will be based on a discussion of the literature on nurse-led surgical clinics, outlining the range and scope of clinics/services, with examples from clinical practice.

Types of nurse-led surgical oncology clinics

From a survey of specialist oncology nurses in the UK there was great variability in the nature of nurses' roles and surgical nurse-led clinics (Farrell 2014). Based on the results of this survey and descriptions in the literature, there seem to be four main types of nurse-led surgical clinics:

- Diagnostic clinics
- Surgical pre-assessment
- Results and minor procedures or dressings after surgery
- Follow-up post-surgery

Diagnostic clinics

There has been an increase in the number of specialist nurses and advanced nurse practitioners working in diagnostic clinics across different cancer groups, however the nature of procedures and investigations undertaken may vary according to each individual and the nature of the clinical environment. Although some nurses may work alongside other clinical/medical colleagues undertaking consultations and diagnostic procedures, other nurses may have their own clinics within the same department. However there is limited evidence in the literature regarding this. An audit of waiting times in a nurse-led diagnostic clinic for post-menopausal bleeding showed that the nurse-led clinic had increased the number of patients meeting the 31-day diagnostic target from 25 per cent (pre-nurse-led clinic) to 82 per cent (post-nurse-led) (Mills 2005).

By the nature of the term itself, diagnostic clinics may involve a number of examinations, investigations and medical procedures before a cancer diagnosis can be established. This can include X-rays, computerised tomography (CT) scans, magnetic resonance imaging (MRI) scans, or specialist scans such as mammography. In addition, a diagnosis of cancer also requires tissue samples to be taken; therefore a biopsy is undertaken of a suspected cancer, which may be conducted at the same clinic appointment. In some cases a fine needle aspiration (FNA) may be undertaken before a biopsy to provide quick interim results of a possible cancer. Nurses are also undertaking nurse-led clinics which include endoscopy (Basnyat et al. 2002), colposcopy, colonoscopy (Farrell et al. 2011) or sigmoidoscopy (Kelly et al. 2008, Maruthachalam et al. 2006).

Nurses may undertake bespoke training to achieve competence in undertaking FNAs and biopsies, however there is little research evidence of this.

Garvican et al. (1998) undertook an audit of 119 FNA investigations in patients with breast cancer attending a nurse-led breast cancer diagnostic clinic, drawing comparisons with FNAs undertaken by doctors. Clinical expertise compared favourably with other clinicians in that nurses produced a lower proportion of inadequate samples, and there was 100 percent satisfaction with clinical care. However only five of the patients seen expected to see a nurse, although being seen by a nurse was acceptable to patients and GPs.

One hundred and twenty patients attending a one-stop nurse-led prostate biopsy clinic reported high satisfaction (Lane and Minns 2010), which reflected similar results from a nurse-led prostate biopsy evaluating 33 patients' experiences (James and McPhail 2008). Although patients were supportive of the nurse-led concept and would not like to see a doctor, 10 per cent said they would have preferred to be seen initially by a consultant urologist (James and McPhail 2008). Satisfaction was similar in a nurse-led bone marrow biopsy clinic, and there was an appropriate quality of samples taken (Collins 2010). In addition, the audit highlighted the benefits of information and support when the procedure was performed by a CNS.

Surgical pre-assessment clinics

The survey of oncology specialist nurses' roles in nurse-led clinics identified that several nurses were undertaking pre-operative assessment clinics; however this was mainly undertaken by nurse practitioners within the research sample (Farrell et al. 2011). There is limited research evidence, which limits understanding of the nature of the role and scope of nurses' practice. However, a study of 12 patients with gynaecological cancer attending a pre-operative assessment clinic, and a further five patients attending a focus group, was undertaken to evaluate the nurse-led clinic (Guest et al. 2012). All patients reported that their needs had been addressed and six (50%) found the holistic needs assessment useful. In addition, the focus group found the nurse-led clinic reassuring, and reported that it provided the opportunity to meet the CNS before surgery, and a platform to discuss any concerns (Guest et al. 2012).

Discussing results and undertaking minor procedures after surgery

An increasing number of specialist nurses are now responsible for giving patients histology results after surgery, across different cancer groups, however there is limited research evidence in the literature regarding this. Twenty patients attending nurse-led clinics for histology results, prior to their medical appointment, reported 100 per cent satisfaction; however patients were not asked whether they would prefer to see a doctor (Warren 2007).

There may be a range of different minor procedures that can be undertaken in a nurse-led surgical clinic, such as aspirating seromas and inflating breast tissue expanders. In addition, nurse-led clinics provide a valuable opportunity for wound care, including dressings (Farrell et al. 2011).

Follow-up post-surgery

The greatest amount of evidence on nurse-led surgical clinics is in relation to nurse-led follow-up after completion of surgery. In some cases the research evaluated the nurse-led clinic; however in some cases studies compared nurse-led and doctor-led care. A large study of 525 patients with breast cancer attending routine follow-up clinics compared nurse versus doctor-led follow-up (Baildam et al. 2004). The findings showed no financial advantage of nurse-led care, and there was no difference in patients' quality of life or psychological distress. However nurses identified psychological distress more frequently than doctors (53% versus 8%). There was also greater satisfaction with nurse-led consultations than medical, although nurses spent a significantly longer time with patients (Baildam et al. 2004).

Five studies focus on nurse-led surgical follow-up clinics for patients with colorectal cancer (McFarlane et al. 2011, Jeyararjah et al. 2010, Knowles 2007, Strand et al. 2011, Wilkinson and Sloane 2009). A feasibility study to assess nurse-led surgical follow-up for 60 patients identified nurse-led follow-up to be safe, efficient and acceptable to patients (Knowles 2007). The study also demonstrated significant improvements in quality of life, and high patient and clinician satisfaction; in addition cost-savings were estimated to be £28,000 per year. Three studies included 950 patients (McFarlane et al. 2011), 121 patients (Wilkinson and Sloan 2009), and 193 patients (Jeyararjah et al. 2010) attending nurse-led follow-up clinics after surgery. Patients reported 95 per cent satisfaction, and high levels of value apportioned to continuity, personalised care and increased ability to discuss their concerns (Wilkinson and Sloan 2009). Decreased costs for nurse-led clinics were reported in comparison to estimates for medical clinics (Jeyararjah et al. 2010); however precise details of cost estimates were not available. One study compared nurse-led and doctor-led follow-up for 110 patients post-surgery for colorectal cancer; demonstrating high levels of patient satisfaction, however nurse consultations were longer (Strand et al. 2011). In addition, more blood samples were taken in nurse-led clinics (29% versus 7%), and surgical assistance was needed in 13 nurse consultations, which had implications for cost estimates. McFarlane et al. (2011) report that the nurse-led follow-up clinic was adjacent to the consultant's clinic, which provided easy access if the CNS had any clinical questions or concerns. Although nurse consultations were longer, this provided greater time for information and education about diet, bowel function, sexual dysfunction and symptoms of recurrence, which may reduce the number and/or frequency of clinic appointments (McFarlane et al. 2011).

Section 4: Nurse-led research clinics

This section will focus on clinical research nurses involved in clinical trials, explaining aspects of their role and implications for clinical practice. I will also discuss the different phases of research studies for clinical trials, and mandatory processes for healthcare research, including ethical and research and development

(R&D) approvals, and informed consent. A discussion of nurse-led clinics for patients on clinical research trials will follow, detailing implications for nurses and clinical practice.

Introduction

Nurses are becoming increasing involved in research within their roles and/or academic courses (Ledger et al. 2008). Although some clinical nurses will undertake academic nursing research as part of their role, this is mainly nurse consultants and to a lesser degree advanced nurse practitioners (ANP) or clinical nurse specialists (CNS) (Farrell et al. 2011). In contrast, the number of research nurses involved in clinical trials has increased rapidly over the last ten years (Spilsbury et al. 2007), and this represents the majority of clinical nurses who are involved in research in NHS hospital trusts.

The importance of research

Research is defined as 'The attempt to produce generalizable new knowledge by addressing clearly defined questions with rigorous and systematic methods' (RCN 2012, p2). The need for evidence-based clinical practice is well recognised, however the majority of clinical research undertaken in the UK is medical research involving clinical trials sponsored by pharmaceutical companies. This is a crucial process in the development of new medicinal products, which takes many years of research and different phases of research in new drug development. In oncology there is a constant drive to develop new anti-cancer drugs and increase the number of patients recruited to clinical trials. Recently this has included a greater emphasis on targeted/biological therapies, which represent novel treatment tailored to individual patients depending on biological aspects of their cancer. The introduction of targeted systemic therapies has had implications for nurses with a steep learning curve to increase their knowledge and understanding so that they can inform patients appropriately. 'As soon as animate feeling beings become the subject of experiment . . . this innocence of the search for knowledge is lost and questions of conscience arise' (Jonas 1969 p2).

Phases of research for clinical trials

When a drug is introduced, the initial studies are done in the laboratory to establish the effects of the drug. Once this toxicology data is obtained and approved, the drug can be tested on humans in the different phases of clinical trials.

There are four phases of clinical trials, however some researchers may have research designs that incorporate two phases of trials in one protocol, for example phases one and two combined, or phase two and three together. This facilitates a seamless transition between the phases of research and may enable the research to be undertaken in less time or with fewer patients.

Phase 1: Human pharmacology

This is used to consider the safety of a drug and the side-effect profile. This is the first time that the drug has been used in humans. A phase one trial may examine new drugs, a new route of administration, a new treatment schedule or dosage. The initial starting dose is determined by pre-clinical trials and toxicology and efficacy data from animal studies. The main aim of a phase one trial is to determine the maximum tolerated dose of the new drug, either alone or in combination with other drugs. The qualitative and quantitative toxicities must also be established. Efficacy is not a goal of phase one trials, hence there is potentially no benefit for the patient, but it may benefit patients in the future. In view of this, benefits and risks must carefully be assessed and explained to the patients.

Phase 2: Exploratory therapeutic

This is used to determine how a treatment works on patients, which may focus on determining the maximum tolerated dose in relation to clinical side-effects and tolerability. Phase two studies determine how effective the drug is on the actual disease. In oncology, the drug is used on specific tumour types, using the established dose from the phase one studies. Endpoints may include identification of toxicities by assessing the side-effects. Severe side-effects could lead to a dose reduction therefore it is important that patients are aware of this prior to consent.

Phase 3: Confirmatory therapeutic

Phase three trials are the most common trials in clinical practice. They are used to test a new treatment against an existing treatment to assess the disease response. The most effective and unbiased way to do this is in a randomised trial, in order to determine whether the observed effect of the new drug is more worthwhile than the standard treatment. This ensures that the results are scientifically valid. In order to further reduce bias blind studies are useful where the doctor is likely to expect differences in toxicities and/or effectiveness.

Phase 4: Therapeutic use

Phase four trials are used when further research is required on licensed products. This may include additional safety data and or to determine side-effects and long term risks/benefits

The number of patients that are required for studies will vary depending on the phase of trial undertaken. For example smaller numbers are recruited to phase one (15–30) and phase two (<100) than phase three (several hundred/thousands) (NCI 2015).

Design of clinical trials

There are several different types of clinical trials, ranging from single subject design to multisite, international trials, which have thousands of participants.

Some of the clinical trials are comparison studies, which involve randomisation to different groups, whilst in some trials patients could receive the same treatment (Berry et al. 1996).

Trials using drug treatments could be open, whereby everyone is aware of the actual drug that the patient is receiving; they could be double-blind, which means that the name of the drug given to the patient is known only to the drug company monitoring and sponsoring the study. An important reason for this being unknown to the patient and clinician, is to eliminate bias when assessing efficacy and toxicities, and is often used when comparing a standard treatment against a new preparation. It is important for comprehension and compliance, that doctors explain this rationale to the patients, prior to seeking their participation in the study.

In addition, the use of placebos in clinical trials is an important consideration with regard to informed consent. The reason for their inclusion in the randomisation, and exact nature of the trial should be emphasised so that patients fully understand that they may receive a placebo as treatment. The use of a placebo is important when assessing the efficacy and toxicity of some treatments, but it is vital that this is explained carefully to patients prior to informed consent.

Randomised trials

The introduction of randomisation in clinical research reduces bias which increases the credibility of the results, and the validity of the study. Passamani (1991) proposes that a properly conducted randomised clinical trial is the best method for both science and ethics. In a randomised clinical trial, a state of clinical equipoise must exist, in that the doctor must be uncertain as to which of the two treatments is the best. This is based on his clinical judgement, and also scientific evidence of the drugs in question.

Stenning (1992) suggests that if a clinician considers that one of the treatments is not appropriate for the patient, entry into a randomised trial would be biased and inappropriate. It should also be ensured that if any interim results of the trial, pertaining to efficacy and toxicity are such that they would affect this state of equipoise, the investigators should be notified, and the trial stopped.

Informed consent

Informed consent is described as 'The process of agreeing to take part in a study based on access to all relevant and easily digestible information about what participation means, in particular in terms of harms and benefits' (RCN 2012, p3). Chapter 4 has already touched on informed consent in relation to autonomy and mental capacity; however this section will provide more detailed explanations, particularly in relation to clinical trials and clinical research nurses. One of the main factors in the process of informed consent is to ensure that people participate freely, without coercion or manipulation, and with sufficient information to enable them to make a fully informed decision about whether to participate in the research. Some patients may worry about saying no in case it has an adverse effect on their future treatment and care, which is not true, therefore it is important that patients are aware of this, even though they may not readily express this worry to clinical staff.

Obtaining fully informed consent is crucial for any participant involved in research. However, there are often greater complexities when the participant is a patient with cancer, given the potential vulnerabilities from the disease and psychological impact. Traditionally, doctors were responsible for obtaining patients' written informed consent and nurses were responsible for providing patients with more detailed information and explaining implications of the proposed treatment/research. With the expansion of nurses' roles and clinical responsibilities this has led to nurses having greater responsibilities within the process of informed consent, including obtaining written informed consent from patients.

Factors essential to informed consent

In UK case law there are three essential requirements for informed consent to be considered valid (RCN 2011):

1. Consent should be given by someone with the mental capacity to do so
2. Participants should have sufficient information to enable an informed decision
3. Consent must be given freely

If any of the above factors cannot be satisfied then the consent is invalid. It is important that nurses are aware of the legal implications within processes of informed consent, particularly regarding mental capacity (Mental Capacity Act Code of Practice 2015, Mental Capacity Act 2005), data protection laws (Boyd 2003, Redsell and Cheater 2001) and research governance (DH 2005).

Ethical implications

To ensure that research is ethically acceptable all research should be subjected to independent scrutiny by a research ethics committee (REC) prior to starting the research. In addition to assessing the research proposal, including aims, outcomes and methods, the ethics committee will carefully consider the participant information sheets and consent forms, seeking reassurance that all participants will be able to freely give informed consent (Smajdor et al. 2009).

From an ethical perspective there are several essential factors that must be included to ensure informed consent and patients' understanding of the proposed research. For example patients must understand the following (RCN 2011):

- The purpose of the research and consent form
- That their consent is voluntary, that they can withdraw at any time without giving a reason and without it compromising their future care

- The potential benefits for them and possible risks from taking part in the research
- What alternative standard treatment is available
- What procedures and investigations are involved, including practical implications of taking part and what will be expected of them
- The duration of the research
- That the research has been approved by a research ethics committee
- How data about them will be handled, stored and used in the study, including for how long after completion of the study.

Patients should also be given written information about the study which details all of the above, including additional written information about the nature of the study/treatment. Contact details should also be provided if patients have further questions, or wish to withdraw from the study. It is also crucial that patients have at least 24 hours to consider the written information before deciding whether to participate in the research, however some patients will require a longer time period for this.

Discussing risks with patients

The General Medical Council (GMC) issued guidance on consent for patients, which included a discussion of assessing risks and conveying information to patients. Information about risks must be clear and accurate and presented in a way that patients can understand. However the variability in information needs is well recognised, therefore information should be tailored to each individual and patient-focused (GMC 2008).

The GMC (2008) defines risks as taking a number of different forms, although in relation to treatments risks usually fall into three main areas:

1. Side-effects
2. Complications
3. Failure of an intervention/treatment to achieve the desired aim

The severity of risks may also vary from minor to serious, and occurrence may vary from common to rare. Serious risks may be perceived as possibility of permanent disability or death. However it is important to provide information about potential risks in a way that is carefully balanced and realistically weighted to convey the potential occurrence to prevent bias and facilitate informed decision-making and consent.

Responsibilities for informed consent

It should also be remembered that informed consent is a process; therefore nurses should ensure that patients are still willing to continue with the study at each visit.

However this is usually done informally unless there are any protocol amendments, in which case the patient may be re-consented.

The overall responsibility for informed consent lies with the lead investigator (also known as the chief investigator or principal investigator). However, the lead researcher (CI) may delegate the task of obtaining informed consent to another individual(s). For this to occur the CI must ensure that delegated others are appropriately trained and competent, which includes specific training in Good Clinical Research Practice DH (2014). The delegation of responsibilities must be clearly documented on a delegation log, where individuals must document their responsibilities within the study along with their signature and date. Awareness of GCP and regulations for research (International Conference on Harmonisation Good Clinical Practice 2015) is crucial. Good Clinical Research Practice is defined as 'A set of internationally recognized ethical and scientific quality requirements which must be observed for designing, conducting, recording and reporting clinical trials that involve the participation of human subjects' (European Directive 2001, Article 1, clause 2).

Types of consent

Legally, oral consent is as good as written consent provided that it can be proven. A consent form only has legal stance if the patient has read it, and then it can only provide evidence of the consent, and lacks legal significance. There are different types of consent:

1. *Expressed consent* is clearly stated by a person, and often is supported by written documentation.
2. *Tacit consent* is assumed but less explicit. It may be part of a 'normal procedure' in that tacit consent can be assumed, therefore, it is usually expressed by a lack of objection to the proposal. For example, a patient going to his general practitioner with a problem allows the doctor to ask questions about it. Similar to this is implicit or implied consent, which is usually inferred from actions, but is not absolute. The notion of tacit consent could, however, become more complicated, for example, a general consent to have blood tests may include an implicit consent to a special blood test, such as HIV. This consent raises ethical problems in view of the psychological and social implications of such a test. In such cases where actual consent is uncertain, this should be clarified with the patient.
3. *Hypothetical consent* is a form of retrospective consent, in that following a medical procedure that the patient wants, the patient is assumed to have consented, even though he had not been asked. This may appear to be relatively straightforward, for example, when the patient is unconscious. However, if the patient is a Jehovah's Witness it raises problems. Hypothetical consent is the least demanding for the patient and gives the most power to the doctor, therefore, the value of the doctor's judgement is an important consideration.

R&D approval processes

In addition to obtaining ethical approval from REC, approval must be obtained from local R&D departments prior to commencing a study within the NHS. If the research will be undertaken at several sites, R&D approval must be obtained from each site. For nurses who are considering undertaking their own research this is an important consideration, since such approvals may take several months and the process may vary according to each R&D department / hospital Trust.

For clinical trials the sponsor and funding body may be the same organisation, for example pharmaceutical companies. However, for nurses undertaking their own research, they are often separate and may incur additional costs, which can vary according to each organisation.

The funding body provides financial support via contracts with individual researchers or their organisation.

The sponsor has responsibility for ensuring that the proposed research design and conduct of the study meet appropriate standards, including quality assurance and monitoring during the study.

The role of the clinical research nurse

Clinical research nurses (CRN) are registered nurses, often at pay band 6 or 7, although some may be working at band 8A or band 5. CRNs in oncology may work within a clinical team, often within one cancer speciality, or within a local/ regional network, or based within a clinical trials unit (Hardicre 2013). The role and responsibilities of CRNs may vary according to each individual, their disease speciality, nature of their clinical trials portfolio and the range of their clinical skills/competencies. However the broad areas of responsibilities include patient recruitment and screening, involvement in informed consent and randomisation, data collection and data recording (Spilsbury et al. 2007). To illustrate the possible variability across salary bands and differences in nurses' autonomy, Gelling (2011) has identified potential differences regarding informed consent (see Table 8.2).

It is clear from the different dimensions of CRNs' roles that nurses face multiple demands (Spilsbury et al. 2007), particularly when trying to coordinate a large number of different clinical trials. However the role of the CRN is poorly understood by other nurses who have not worked alongside them, which is particularly true of some ward-based nurses (Spilsbury et al. 2007). This may lead to problems for patients, and research nurses, if clinical procedures and management are not followed appropriately in accordance with the clinical trial protocols, or where patients are admitted to hospital and the clinical research team are not informed. Although some clinical trials may be quite straightforward in terms of treatment and clinical management, others can be very complex. This may be due to the randomisation procedures, treatment regimens, pharmacodynamics or requirements for patient investigations and follow-up schedules.

In recent years some of the responsibility of data documentation and organisation has devolved to data managers and clinical trial coordinators, which has

Table 8.2 Clinical research nurses' roles in informed consent (Gelling 2011)

Band 5	Band 6	Band 7	Band 8
• Contact with research participants to ensure understanding of information. • Recognises that informed consent is an ongoing process. • Demonstrates awareness of factors contributing to autonomous decision-making during the consent process. • Complies with informed consent processes within approved protocols, including using approved versions of patient information sheets and consent forms. • Raises any concerns about informed consent processes. • Recognises own learning needs and takes responsibility for maintaining up to date knowledge. • Provides evidence of training and understanding.	• Demonstrates a sound understanding of the need to identify issues which may impact on the process of gaining valid informed consent. • Plans and implements actions to resolve these issues. • Receives informed consent when appropriate and as agreed in the approved protocol. • Supports participants through the consent process.	• Acts as an expert resource to provide in-depth knowledge on aspects pertinent to acquiring and maintaining informed consent. • Contributes to the mentorship and monitoring of consent procedures. • Responsible for the reporting of poor consent processes that compromise patient safety and the study protocol.	Demonstrates leadership by: • Attending and reporting to corporate boards regarding governance, policy and service development related to research. • Holding responsibility for the training and monitoring of correct consent processes in research. • Developing systems to ensure that correct procedures are adhered to. • Contributing to the professional development and education of clinical research staff in the organisation.

reduced some of the paperwork that nurses must complete for each study. Nurses work very closely with the principle investigators for each trial to ensure each trial runs smoothly, maintaining safe conduct and strict adherence to the trial protocols (Hardicre 2013).

Nurse-led clinics for patients on clinical trials

Winter et al. (2012) suggest that a competency framework, from novice to expert, can be utilised for clinical research nurses, which incorporates history-taking, physical examination and non-medical prescribing in stages from proficiency levels 3–5. This type of framework would be useful to assess nurses' skills and competencies over time, and could also provide guidance for nurses seeking to develop nurse-led clinics.

The scope for nurse-led research clinics depends on a number of different factors; however this may be compromised by regulations from individual pharmaceutical companies. Similarly, this can have an adverse effect on nurses' roles within advanced nursing practice. When clinical trials are being set up there are extensive discussions between pharmaceutical companies and clinicians (medical consultants and CRNs) to ensure that the requirements for each trial can be met within standard clinical practice. When conducting the trial clinicians must ensure that all mandatory assessments are undertaken at the appropriate time and by an appropriate clinician.

The delegation of clinical duties within a trial is documented in a delegation log, which provides a signed record of each person's responsibilities. The introduction of advanced practice nursing roles has created some difficulties where their clinical skills and responsibilities are neither understood, nor recognised by some pharmaceutical companies, which can place limitations on the scope of nurses' practice within clinical trials. Therefore it is important to seek approval from each company or principal investigator to enable ANPs to conduct medical examinations for all clinical trials. This is easier during the early stages of negotiations when setting up clinical trials, than trying to achieve it after commencement of a trial.

I found this very frustrating when I was a nurse clinician since it created disparities in practice. For example in some clinical trials I could undertake full clinical examination, history-taking and prescribing, whilst in other trials I was not allowed to examine patients since they required a doctor to do this, and not a nurse with the same level of clinical skills. This also restricted my ability to set up some nurse-led clinics for patients on clinical trials, which could have improved the efficiency of service delivery and continuity for patients. Therefore the scope of nurses' roles and opportunities to develop nurse-led research clinics is determined and restricted by specifications within the trial protocol. However, we can often work with this and be creative with different models of nurse-led practice.

Different models of nurse-led clinics

When developing nurse-led clinics it is crucial to adopt a team approach and consider the skill mix of individuals within the team, since this can be used to create different levels of nurse-led clinics.

During my own clinical practice as a nurse clinician I worked closely with the clinical research nurses to streamline patient care within clinical trials and provide greater continuity. At the cancer centre there are patients on phase two or three clinical trials of intravenous SACT, including novel unlicensed drugs, therefore it is the CRN's responsibility to administer the treatment and carefully monitor patients during this process. This may also involve additional research procedures, such as nursing assessments, observations at specific time points, electrocardiographs (ECGs), and taking additional blood tests for trial purposes, including pharmacokinetics/pharmacodynamics. All of this can be undertaken within a nurse-led service which clearly highlights the autonomy of nurses' roles. This is enhanced if nurses have their own clinic rooms and treatment beds within existing locations, or within a designated clinical trials unit. However this model of nurse-led clinic relies on other clinical staff to undertake clinical/medical assessments/examinations and prescribing. This may also include ordering further investigations; however some CRNs will have extended responsibilities to undertake this within their current role.

The next level of nurse-led research clinics involves clinical consultations with some patients that they can undertake independently from medical staff. For example a CRN would often work with me in my nurse-led chemotherapy clinic to assess patients during treatment, including chemotherapy toxicities and data collection required for trial purposes. They could see patients independently during treatment and I would prescribe the chemotherapy and other medicines. However, if patients were unwell I could see and examine them and make the appropriate clinical decisions. This use of skill mix and close liaison worked very well, reducing patient waiting time and ensured appropriate collection of trial data. It also facilitated recruitment to clinical trials since the CRNs and I worked together with new patients; they would discuss information about the trial, including implications and I would obtain written informed consent alongside them. The CRNs and I also worked together in the follow-up of patients on clinical trials when patients on adjuvant clinical trials attended my nurse-led follow-up clinics. I would undertake the clinical consultation and physical examination and the research nurses would collect additional data required for trial purposes and ensure that timing of the next appointment was appropriate. However, given my understanding of the CRN role, having undertaken this in the past and continuing to work closely with the research nurses, I was also able to collect the required trial data if the CRNs were busy elsewhere in the hospital.

The final model of nurse-led care represents the highest level of nurse-led clinic where CRNs have responsibility for episodes of clinical management, independent from medical staff. This requires the skills of an advanced nurse practitioner who is able to undertake clinical examinations, history-taking, non-medical prescribing, obtain written informed consent, order investigations and interpret the results, and make clinical decisions within the remit of the trial protocols. This nurse-led clinic could run independently from, or in parallel to, the medical clinics. However a parallel clinic would enable nurses to practice autonomously yet have easy access to medical colleagues if required. Table 8.3 illustrates different levels of nurse-led research clinics, based on my own practice.

Section 5: Nurse-led follow-up clinics

There are many examples of models of care for routine cancer follow-up. This section will discuss different models of nurse-led clinics, including telephone

Table 8.3 Different levels of nurse-led research clinics

Level	Role and responsibilities
Level 1	• Clinical trial data collection • Nursing assessments, observations and obtain blood samples • Administer systemic treatments as per trial protocols
Level 2	Level 1 responsibilities plus: • Undertake basic clinical consultations with patients in liaison with a clinician • Order investigations
Level 3	Level 2 responsibilities plus: • Undertake independent clinical consultations with patients in liaison with a clinician • Obtain written informed consent • Order investigations independently • Interpret the results of investigations and liaise with a clinician • Non-medical prescribing
Level 4	Level 3 responsibilities plus: • Undertake independent clinical consultations and history-taking • Undertake comprehensive clinical examinations • Autonomous clinical decision-making in accordance with trial protocols, and liaison with medical consultant / principal investigator

nurse-led clinics, shared care protocols and fully autonomous nurse-led follow-up clinics. In addition, there will be a discussion of the evidence-base and rationale for routine cancer follow-up, survivorship initiatives and programmes that have influenced clinical practice developments.

Literature on nurse-led follow-up

Two literature reviews of 11 and 37 studies respectively (Cusack and Taylor 2010; Cox and Wilson 2003) indicate that telephone consultations are an appropriate means of providing nurse-led follow-up. In particular telephone follow-up for patients with colorectal cancer is considered to be cost-effective and accepted by the majority of patients (Cusack and Taylor 2010); aspects of care include symptom management and also highlight the potential to provide reassurance over the phone.

This highlights how services are changing to meet increasing demands in the medical clinics, and also how nurses are being used to address this. The majority of nurse-led telephone clinics are used to replace routine follow-up after early treatment, which was previously undertaken in outpatient clinics by doctors. An indication of the interest in telephone clinics is illustrated by the number of studies using this method for a range of cancer groups including prostate cancer (Booker et al. 2004; Helgessen et al. 2000), ovarian cancer (Cox et al. 2008), lung cancer (Lewis et al. 2009; Moore et al. 2006; Corner 2003; Moore et al. 2002), and breast cancer (Kimman et al. 2011, 2010; Beaver et al. 2010, 2009, 2006; Sheppard et al. 2009; Koinberg et al. 2004, 2002; Brown et al. 2002).

All nurse-led clinics appear to score highly on patient satisfaction surveys, and although some patients seem to prefer the reassurance of traditional clinic follow-up, this appears to be a small minority (Lewis et al. 2009). A difference in patients' expectations may create some natural resistance in the early stages of developing nurse-led clinics and changing from traditional clinics, particularly if patients are uncertain about nurses' roles (Fitzsimmons et al. 2005). However over a period of time the concept of nurse-led clinics may become more acceptable to patients as the normal method of follow-up. Nevertheless it appears that patients do not have much, if any, choice in the method of follow-up outside of research studies.

Beaver et al. (2006) conducted a randomised trial to compare standard doctor-led follow-up with nurse-led telephone follow-up using an intervention to address information needs (Beaver et al. 2009). However, this approach creates a very structured nurse-led consultation. In contrast the approach in other nurse-led telephone clinics is less structured when focusing on information and symptom management (Kimman et al. 2010; Cox et al. 2008; Booker et al. 2004).

A number of studies place more responsibility on patients themselves during routine follow-up by using a nurse-led telephone service on demand for patients with prostate cancer (Helgessen et al. 2000), or patient-initiated follow-up after breast cancer (Sheppard et al. 2009; Koinberg et al. 2004, 2002; Brown et al. 2002). Although on demand services are considered safe, acceptable and convenient, some patients seem to prefer the reassurance of a clinical examination, therefore patient choice seems an important consideration.

In summary there is strong evidence from research studies that nurse-led clinics are acceptable to patients, irrespective of the mode of delivery, however patient choice is important. Although telephone follow-up is safe, effective and acceptable to the majority of patients, some will prefer attending clinics where they can have a face-to-face discussion. The potential benefits of involving patients in nurse-led service developments is clear (Fitzsimmons et al. 2005), however this study also demonstrates patients' lack of understanding regarding expansion to nurses' traditional roles, and illustrates how this may influence their acceptance of nurse-led clinics.

Different models of nurse-led care

In follow-up clinics where nurses have replaced the doctor, the nurses' role appears to follow a medical model of care: checking for possible recurrence, checking for signs and symptoms and undertaking a clinical examination (Baildam et al. 2004; Strand et al. 2011). Similarly, swapping a medical clinic for nurse-led telephone clinic may also be conducted in a structured way to elicit signs or symptoms of possible recurrence (Brown et al. 2002; Koinberg et al. 2002, 2004; Knowles 2007; Sheppard et al. 2009; Kimman et al. 2011) or side-effects of treatment (Booker et al. 2004).

In contrast, some of the nurse-led follow-up clinics set out to provide something different, or additional to, the medical clinics. After identifying problems within the medical clinic for patients with lung cancer, the nurse-led clinic was set up to focus on the patient as a whole, trying to improve complex symptoms and coordinate care (Corner et al. 2002; Moore et al. 2002; Moore et al. 2006). This new model of nurse-led care provided significant benefits for patients, including increased satisfaction, improved symptom management, reduced dyspnoea, improved emotional functioning, and fewer medical appointments, and patients were more likely to die at home than hospital or hospice (Corner et al. 2002; Moore et al. 2002). Moore et al. (2006) demonstrated greater contact with palliative care teams, improved psychosocial and financial support and improved coordination of care from nurse-led clinics.

Despite frequent suggestions in the literature that nurse-led clinics can offer advantages to patients by undertaking holistic care, or by offering psychological support, there is little evidence of this taking place. There are no details of nurses' consultations with patients within nurse-led clinics, and minimal descriptions of nurses' roles, which creates speculation regarding the nature and content of consultations and nurse-patient interactions.

Symptom management

A literature review of 11 studies focuses on telephone follow-up after surgery for colorectal cancer where symptom management is successfully undertaken and provides reassurance for patients (Cusack and Taylor 2010). In these studies telephone follow-up is undertaken by specialist nurses who are familiar with the common symptoms and able to discuss strategies over the phone to improve patients' symptoms, for example nutrition and diet to alleviate bowel problems.

For patients with lung cancer, symptom management appears complex and nurse-led clinics adopt an alternative approach (Corner et al. 2002; Moore et al. 2002). The authors identify that dyspnoea is a complex symptom, incorporating psychological, physical and physiological elements, which requires an alternative approach to standard medical reviews or doctor-nurse substitution. Patients are taught different breathing and relaxation techniques, psychosocial and financial concerns are addressed, the disease monitored, symptoms managed and care coordinated through the nurse-led clinics and liaison with palliative care services. A combination of face-to-face clinics and telephone clinics are used, with a patient-centred approach tailored to each individual (Corner et al. 2002; Moore et al. 2002).

Policy influences on clinical management

Current cancer policies emphasise the need for change and to develop innovative ways of working. In the Cancer Reform Strategy (DH 2007), the need for flexibility within the NHS to meet patients' needs and introduce greater choices for patients is directly linked with developing nurses' roles and models of nurse-led care.

Despite legislation not keeping pace with clinical developments, there has been a huge drive for nurses to develop their roles, with a significant increase in nurse-led clinics and services. Although financial constraints in the NHS, together with a reduction in junior medical staff, may influence the development of nurse-led services, there may be a similar drive from nurses themselves.

Clinical developments influencing nurse-led clinics

As discussed throughout this chapter there is an increased prevalence of nurse-led clinics for routine follow-up. The drive for such nurse-led clinics has mainly been influenced by increasing clinical demands. For example government targets in relation to waiting times for new referrals/commencement of treatment post cancer diagnosis regularly resulted in the deferral or cancellation of routine follow-up appointments and/or medical clinics exceeding capacity. Therefore the management of patients on routine follow-up was devolved to specialist nurses. In many cases nurse-led follow-up clinics were set up in a rush to meet clinical demands, therefore nurses' clinical skills may have restricted what they were able to do within nurse-led clinics:

- If clinical examination is required within nurse-led follow-up clinics, nurses must undertake additional training in order to do this competently. Where nurses are working within one disease group, such as breast cancer, they may only need to be competent to undertake breast examination, since the need to undertake respiratory, cardiovascular and abdominal examinations would be rare. However if nurses are working with complex patients or across several cancer groups they may need more comprehensive clinical examination skills to meet patients' needs.
- If investigations are required within nurse-led follow-up, nurses must be able to order these independently, interpret the results, inform patients and discuss the results with them. However, if there are indications of disease progression nurses must liaise with medical colleagues to discuss further management, therefore systems must be in place to support this in a timely manner.
- If medicines need to be prescribed within nurse-led follow-up nurses must either be independent non-medical prescribers, or have systems in place to delegate prescribing to a hospital clinician or the patient's GP. For example, patients with breast cancer on endocrine treatment may be managed in nurse-led follow-up by nurses who do or do not prescribe, since any changes required to endocrine treatment can be managed by writing to the patient's GP. If such treatment needs to start or change urgently, the letter can be faxed to reduce waiting time. This system may seem appropriate for occasional use, however if medicines regularly need to be prescribed within nurse-led clinics it is better if the nurse is an independent prescriber.

In order for nurse-led follow-up clinics to run efficiently and effectively, there should be careful consideration of clinical responsibilities to determine what clinical skills are essential and desirable. Protocols and operational policies should be put in place to ensure transparency with the scope of nurses' roles and boundaries of clinical practice. However, protocols may change over time with further developments to nurses' roles and nurse-led clinics.

The infrastructure of the nurse-led clinic should also be considered prior to set up, including room allocation, administrative and secretarial support. It is also crucial to arrange cover for the nurse-led clinic from another nurse with similar training and experience, or a medical colleague; however they must be familiar with operational aspects of your nurse-led clinic to ensure consistency for patients.

Summary

The debate continues around nurse-led clinics regarding whether advanced practice is doctor-nurse substitution or an extension of nurses' existing roles, although the literature review demonstrates acceptability for patients and effective clinical outcomes with nurse-led clinics. Furthermore, several studies report the 'added value' of nurse-led care in providing a more holistic package of care for patients than simply nurse-doctor substitution. Clearly in oncology there has been a rapid increase in the number and nature of nurse-led clinics and services over the past decade, which reflects the changes in government and professional policies, the advances in non-medical prescribing, and influences by nurses and patients themselves. However, despite such advances in nurse-led service provision, this is mainly in relation to follow-up care within oncology.

The variability in chemotherapy provision in the UK presents an increasing challenge in view of limitations in capacity and resources at cancer centres and units, which leads to greater consideration for nurse-led models of care in relation to chemotherapy administration and clinical management of patients in outpatient departments. Although this creates a great potential for nurses to develop their practice and set up nurse-led clinics, it is important to ensure that adequate training, preparation and support for such posts are provided to keep pace with professional and clinical developments.

One explanation for the increased prevalence of nurse-led follow-up clinics may be because the clinical management of patients on routine follow-up is more straightforward than patients who receive chemotherapy or radiotherapy treatment. Patients on follow-up require less input from medical staff and prescribing is infrequent, which increases nurses' independence. In contrast, patients receiving chemotherapy or radiotherapy are more likely to have medical problems during treatment that are beyond the scope of some specialist nurses; clinical decision-making is more complex, and a higher level of clinical skills is often required.

With the current emphasis on survivorship and changes in follow-up care provision, specialist nurses can play a key role in improving patients' experiences, their quality of life, psychosocial well-being and communication as well as cancer surveillance. The development and standardisation of advanced roles and associated educational preparation is important when taking forward the survivorship agenda and developing appropriate pathways for follow-up care given the current shift to nurse-led follow-up in many areas. Nurses are in a prime position to provide holistic assessments, continuity and ease of access whilst tailoring follow-up care to each individual, and this seems an important consideration given the current drive in the UK of moving cancer care away from tertiary centres into primary care and closer to home for patients.

References

Baildam A, Keeling F, Thompson L, Bundred N, Hopwood P. (2004). Nurse-led surgical follow-up clinics for women treated for breast cancer – a randomised controlled trial. *European Journal of Cancer*. 38 (Suppl. 3): S136–137.

Basnyat P, Gomez K, West J, Davies P, Foster M. (2002). Nurse-led direct access endoscopy clinics. *Eco Health*. 16: 166–169.

Beaver K, Williamson S, Chalmers K. (2010). Telephone follow up after treatment for breast cancer: views and experiences of patients and specialist breast care nurses. *Journal of Clinical Nursing*. 19(19–20): 2916–2924.

Beaver K, Tysver-Robinson D, Campbell M, Twomey M, Williamson S, Hindley A, Susnerwala S, Dunn G, Luker K. (2009). Comparing hospital and telephone follow up after treatment for breast cancer: randomised equivalence trial. *British Medical Journal*. 338: 3147–3156.

Beaver K, Twomey M, Witham G, Foy S, Luker K. (2006). Meeting the information needs of women with breast cancer: Piloting a nurse-led intervention. *European Journal of Oncology Nursing*. 10: 378–390.

Berry DL, Dodd MJ, Hinds PS, Ferrell BR. (1996). Informed Consent: Process and Clinical Issues. *Oncology Nursing Forum*. 23(3): 507–512.

Booker J, Eardley A, Cowan R, Logue J, Wylie J, Caress AL. (2004). Telephone first post-intervention follow up for men who have had radical radiotherapy to the prostate: evaluation of a novel service delivery approach. *European Journal of Oncology Nursing*. 8(4): 325–333.

Boyd P. (2003). The requirements of the Data Protection Act 1998 for the processing of medical data. *Journal of Medical Ethics*. 29(1), 34–35.

Brown L, Payne S, Royle G. (2002). Patient initiated follow up of breast cancer. *Psycho-Oncology*. 11: 346–355.

Campbell J, German L, Lane C. (1999). Radiotherapy outpatient review: a nurse-led clinic. *Nursing Standard*. 13(22): 39–44.

Collins J. (2010). Audit of a nurse-led bone marrow biopsy clinic. *Cancer Nursing Practice*. 9(4): 14–19.

Corner J (2003). The role of nurse-led care in cancer management. *Lancet Oncology*. 4(10): 631–636

Cox A, Bull E, Cockle-Hearne J, Knibb W, Potter C, Faithfull S. (2008). Nurse led telephone follow up in ovarian cancer: A psychosocial perspective. *European Journal of Oncology Nursing*. 12(5): 412–417.

Cox K, Wilson E. (2003). Follow up for people with cancer: nurse-led services and telephone interventions. *Journal of Advanced Nursing*. 43(1): 51–61.

Cusack M, Taylor C. (2010). A literature review of the potential of follow up in colorectal cancer. *Journal of Clinical Nursing*. 19(17–8): 2394–2405.

Department of Health. (2003). *Strengthening the accountability, policy and practical guidance for section 11 Health and Social care act (2001)*. London, Department of Health.

Department of Health. (2005). *Research governance framework for health and social care*, 2nd ed. London, Department of Health.

Department of Health. (2007). *The cancer reform strategy*. London, Department of Health.

Department of Health. (2009). Impact assessment of national chemotherapy advisory group recommendations. Available at: http//tinyurl.com/8a7pfyq [accessed 25.03.2012].

DH. (2014). Good clinical practice for clinical trials. Avaliable at: https://www.gov.uk/good-clinical-practice-for-clinical-trials [last accessed 29.07.2015].

Earnshaw J, Stephenson Y. (1997). First two years of a follow up breast clinic led by a nurse practitioner. *Journal of the Royal Society of Medicine*. 90: 258–259.

Egan M, Dowling M. (2005). Patients' satisfaction with a nurse-led oncology service. *British Journal of Nursing*. 14(21): 1112–1116.

European Directive. (2001). Available at: http://ec.europa.eu/health/human-use/clinical-trials/index_en.htm [accessed 16.02.2015].

Faithfull S, Corner J, Meyer L, Huddart R, Dearnaley D. (2001). Evaluation of a nurse-led follow up for patients undergoing pelvic radiotherapy. *British Journal of Cancer*. 85(12): 1853–1864.

Faithfull S, Hunt G. (2005). Exploring nursing values in the development of a nurse-led service. *Nursing Ethics*. 12(5): 440–452.

Farrell C. (2014). *An exploration of oncology nurse specialists' roles in nurse-led chemotherapy clinics*. Unpublished PhD thesis, University of Manchester.

Farrell C, Molassiotis A, Beaver K, Heaven C. (2011). Exploring the scope of oncology specialist nurses' practice in the UK. *European Journal of Oncology Nursing*. 15(2): 160–166.

Fitzsimmons D, Hawker SE, Simmonds P, George SL, Johnson CD, Corner JL. (2005). Nurse-led models of chemotherapy care: mixed economy or nurse-doctor substitution. *Journal of Advanced Practice*. 50(3): 244–252.

Fletcher J, Hornsby C. (2007). Radiotherapy review for patients with breast cancer: a new approach. *Cancer Nursing Practice*. 6(4): 35–39.

Garvican L, Grimsey E, Littlejohns P, Lownds S, Sacks N. (1998). Satisfaction with clinical nurse specialists in breast care clinic: questionnaire survey. *BMJ* 316: 976–977.

Gelling L. (2011). *Competency framework for clinical research nurses*. http://www.crn.nihr.ac.uk/wp-content/uploads/Learning%20and%20development/Research%20Nurse%20Competency%20Framework-Oct2011.pdf

General Medical Council. (2008). *Consent: patients and doctors making decisions together*. Available at: http://www.gmc-uk.org/guidance/ethical_guidance/consent_guidance_index.asp [accessed 16.02.2015].

Gerrish K, Lacey A. (2010). *The research process in nursing*, 6th ed. Oxford, Wiley and Sons.

Good Clinical Practice. (n.d.). Available at: www.mhra.gov.uk/Howweregulate/Medicines/Inspectionandstandards/GoodClinicalPractice [accessed 16.02.2015].

Guest A, Manderville H, Thompson R. (2012). Developing a clinic to meet patient's pre-operative needs. *Cancer Nursing Practice*. 11(3): 25–29.

Hardicre J. (2013). An exploration of the role of the research nurse and its impact. *British Journal of Nursing*. 22(3): 168–169.

Helgessen F, Andersson SO, Gustafsson O, Varenhorst E, Gobén B, Carnock S, Sehlstedt L, Carlsson P, Holmberg L, Johansson JE. (2000). Follow-up of prostate cancer patients by on-demand contacts with a specialist nurse: a randomized Study. *Scandinavian Journal of Urology and Nephrology*. 34(1): 55–61.

International Conference on Harmonisation Good Clinical Practice. (1996). Available at: http://ichgcp.net/ [accessed 16.02.2015].

James N, McPhail G. (2008). The success of a nurse-led, one stop suspected prostate cancer clinic. *Cancer Nursing Practice*. 7: 3, 28–32.

Jeyarajah S, Adams KJ, Higgins L, Ryan S, Leather AJ, Papagrigoriadis S. (2010). Prospective evaluation of a colorectal cancer nurse follow-up clinic. *Colorectal Disease*. 13(1): 31–38.

Jonas H. (1969). Daedalus. *Journal of the American Academy of arts and Science*. Spring edition: 219–246.

Kelly SB, Murphy J, Smith A, Watson H, Gibb S, Walker C, Reddy R. (2008). Nurse specialist led flexible sigmoidoscopy in an outpatient setting. *Colorectal Disease*. 10(4): 390–393.

Kimman ML, Bloebaum MM, Dirksen CD, Houben RM. (2010). Patient satisfaction with nurse-led telephone follow up after curative treatment for breast cancer. *BMC Cancer*. 10: 174.

Kimman ML, Dirksen CD, Voogd, C, Falger P, Gijsen BC, Thuring M, Lenssen A, van der Ent F, Verkeyn J, Haekens C, Hupperets P, Nuytinck JK, vanRiet Y, Brenninkmeijer SJ, Scheijmans LJ, Kessels A, Lambin P, Boersma LJ. (2011). Nurse-led telephone follow-up and an educational group programme after breast cancer treatment: results of a 2 x 2 randomised controlled trial. *European Journal of Cancer*. 47(7): 1027–1036.

Knowles G. (2007). *Advanced nursing practice framework – Cancer nurse specialist example*. Report prepared for the Scottish Government. Available at: http://www.advanced-practice.scot.nhs.uk/media/1282/appendix_1a__1.the_toolkit_concept__1.1overview.pdf [accessed 23.05.2015].

Koinberg IL, Fridlund B, Engholm GB, Holmberg L. (2004). Nurse-led follow up on demand or by a physician after breast cancer surgery: a randomised study. *European Journal of Oncology Nursing*. 8(2): 109–117; discussion 118–120.

Koinberg IL, Holmberg L, Fridlund B. (2002). Breast cancer patients' satisfaction with a spontaneous system of check-up visits to a specialist nurse. *Scandinavian Journal of Caring Science*. 16: 209–215.

Lane L, Minns S. (2010). Empowering advanced nurse practitioners to set up nurse-led clinics for improved outpatient care. *Nursing Times.net*. Available at: http://www.nursingtimes.net/nursing-practice/specialisms/practice-nursing/empowering-advanced-practitioners-to-set-up-nurse-led-clinics-for-improved-outpatient-care/5013288.article [accessed 16.02.15].

Ledger T, Pulfrey A, Luke J. (2008). Developing clinical research nurses. *Nursing Management*. 15(2): 28–33.

Lee H, Lim Y, Yoo MS, Kim Y. (2011). Effects of a nurse-led cognitive behaviour therapy on fatigue and quality of life in patients with breast cancer undergoing radiotherapy: an exploratory study. *Cancer Nursing*. 34(6): 22–30.

Lennan E, McPhelim J. (2012). A snapshot of innovation: chemotherapy delivery in the UK. *British Journal of Nursing*. 21(4): S12–15.

Lewis R, Neal RD, Williams NH, France B, Wilkinson C, Hendry M, Russell D, Russell I, Hughes DA, Stuart NSA, Weller D. (2009). Nurse-led vs. conventional physician-ed follow up for patients with cancer: systematic review. *Journal of Advanced Nursing*. 65(4): 706–723.

Maruthachalam K, Stoker E, Nicholson G, Horgan A. (2006). Nurse-led flexible sigmoidoscopy in primary care – the first thousand patients. *Colorectal Disease*. 8: 557–562.

McFarlane K, Dixon L, Wakeman CJ, Robertson GM, Eglinton TW, Frizelle FA. (2011). The process and outcomes of a nurse-led colorectal cancer follow-up clinic. *Colorectal Disease*. 14: e245–249.

Mental Capacity Act. (2005). Available at: www.legislation.gov.uk/ukpga/2005/9/contents [accessed 16.02.2015].

Mental Capacity Act Code of Practice. (2015). Available at: www.justice.gov.uk/downloads/protecting-the-vulnerable/mca-code-practice-0509.pdf [accessed 16.02.2015].

Mills S. (2005). Reducing waiting times in diagnosing patients with endometrial cancer. *Cancer Nursing Practice*. 4(9): 34–35.

Moore S, Corner J, Haviland J, Wells M, Salmon E, Normand C, Brada M, O'Brien M, Smith I. (2002). Nurse led follow up and conventional medical follow up in management of patients with lung cancer: randomised trial. *British Medical Journal*. 325 (7373): 1145–1147.

Moore S, Wells M, Plant H, Fuller F, Wright M, Corner J. (2006). Nurse specialist led follow up in lung cancer: the experience of developing and delivering a new model of care. *European Journal of Oncology Nursing*. 10(5): 364–377.

National Cancer Institute. (2009). *Common Terminology Criteria for Adverse Events. Version 4*. National Cancer Institute. Available at: http://evs.nci.nih.gov/ftp1/CTCAE/Archive/CTCAE_4.02_2009-09-15_QuickReference_8.5x11.pdf [accessed 23.05.2015].

National Cancer Institute (NCI). (2015). *Phases of clinical trials*. Available at: http://www.cancer.gov/clinicaltrials/learningabout/what-are-clinical-trials/phases [accessed 16.02.2015].

National Chemotherapy Advisory Group. (2009). *Chemotherapy services in England: Ensuring quality and safety. A report from the National Chemotherapy Advisory Group*. London, Department of Health.

NCEPOD. (2008). *For better, for worse? A review of the care of patients who died within 30 days of receiving systemic anti-cancer therapy*. London, NCEPOD.

Nursing and Midwifery Council. (2015). *The Code: Professional standards of practice and behaviour for nurses and midwives*. London, NMC.

Passamani E. (1991). 'Clinical trials – are they ethical?' *New England Journal of Medicine* 324(22): 1589–1591.

Redsell SA, Cheater FM. (2001). The Data Protection Act (1998): implications for health researchers. *Journal of Advanced Nursing*. 35(4), 508–513.

Royal College of Nursing. (2011). *Informed consent in health and social care research: RCN guidance for nurses*. London, RCN.

Royal College of Nursing. (2012). *Informed consent in healthcare research: RCN guidance for nurses* (2nd ed.). London, RCN.

Seibaek L, Petersen LK. (2009). Nurse-led rehabilitation after gynaecological cancer surgery: provisional results from a clinically controlled prospective questionnaire study. *Supportive Care in Cancer*. 17(5): 601–605.

Sharp L, Tishelman C. (2005). Smoking cessation for patients with head and neck cancer: A qualitative study of patients' and nurses' experiences in a nurse-led intervention. *Cancer Nursing*. 28(3): 226–235.

Sheppard C, Higgins B, Wise M, Yiangou C, Dubois D, Kilburn S. (2009). Breast cancer follow up: a randomised controlled trial comparing point of need access versus routine 6-monthly clinical review. *European Journal of Oncology Nursing*. 13: 2–8.

Smajdor A, Sydes MR, Gelling L, Wilkinson M. (2009). Applying for ethical approval for research in the United Kingdom. *British Medical Journal*. 339: 968–972.

Spilsbury K, Petherick E, Cullum N, Nelson A, Nixon J, Mason S. (2007). The role and potential contribution of clinical research nurses to clinical trials. *Journal of Clinical Nursing*. 17(4), 549–557.

Stenning S. (1992). The uncertainty principle: selection of patients for cancer clinical trials. In *Introducing New Treatments for Cancer: Practical, Ethical and Legal Problems* (CJ Williams, ed.) pp. 160–172. Chichester, John Wiley and Sons.

Strand E, Nygren I, Bergkvist L, Smedh K. (2011). Nurse or surgeon follow up after rectal cancer: a randomized trial. *Colorectal Disease*. 13(9): 999–1003.

Vickers E, Uzzell M, Burnet K. (2012). Understanding how targeted therapies work. *Cancer Nursing Practice*. 11(7): 14–22.

Warren M. (2007). Breast cancer patient satisfaction with the nurse-led clinic for surgical histology. *Cancer Nursing Practice*. 6(7): 35–39.

Wells M, Donnan PT, Sharp L, Ackland C, Fletcher J, Dewar JA. (2008). A study to evaluate nurse-led on treatment review for patients undergoing radiotherapy for head and neck cancer. *Journal of Clinical Nursing*. 17(11): 1428–1439.

Wilkinson S, Sloan K. (2009). Patient satisfaction with colorectal cancer follow-up system: an audit. *British Journal of Nursing*. 18(1): 40–44.

Winter H, Lavender V, Blesing C. (2012). Developing a nurse-led clinic for patients enrolled in clinical trials. *Cancer Nursing Practice*. 10(3): 20–24.

Wiseman T, Verity R, Ream E, Alderman E, Richardson A. (2005). *Exploring the work of nurses who administer chemotherapy: A multi-methods study*. London, King's College London.

Chapter 9

Nurse-led pathway for patients with HER2 positive breast cancer receiving Trastuzumab (Herceptin)

Helen Roe

This chapter provides an in-depth case study of a nurse-led clinic. It focuses on the development, implementation, ongoing evaluation and latest update of a nurse-led pathway for Human Epidermal Growth Factor Receptor 2 (HER2) positive breast cancer patients receiving Trastuzumab (Herceptin). Although the primary focus was on early-stage disease, the pathway also includes some patients with metastatic disease. The various stages of the pathway development will be explained and supported by relevant evidence from the appropriate time period.

Background information

Trastuzumab is a recombinant humanised IgG1 monoclonal antibody that targets the HER2, and is used to treat breast (and gastric) cancers where the cancer over expresses HER2. Such patients are generally referred to as HER2 positive (HER2+) (Roche, 2006). Patients with HER2+ breast cancer were thought to account for approximately 15 to 25 per cent of all breast cancer patients, and this cancer associated with an aggressive-behaving tumour, leading to a worse prognosis for the patient (Piccart-Gebhart et al., 2005).

A national decrease in the mortality rate for breast cancer was thought to be due to early detection as a result of the national screening programme in England and Wales since 1988 and advancements in treatment options (National Statistics, 2005) such as Trastuzumab. Trastuzumab was introduced in 2006 for HER2 positive early breast cancer and required all patients to be tested to determine if they were eligible to receive the drug as part of their treatment (National Cancer Research Institute [NCRI] Breast Clinical Studies Group, 2005).

Although the national incidence of breast cancer had increased, fewer people were dying as a result of breast cancer, and for patients diagnosed nationally between 1998 and 2001 the approximate five-year survival rate was around 80 per cent (Quinn, 2005). Clinical trials for patients with HER2+ breast cancer in the adjuvant setting had shown significant benefits in overall disease-free survival from the administration of Trastuzumab for 12 months post chemotherapy (Piccart-Gebhart et al., 2005) The results were so compelling that adjuvant Trastuzumab was quickly introduced into standard clinical practice.

The National Institute of Clinical Excellence (NICE, 2006a) issued its guidance regarding the use of Trastuzumab earlier than expected due to the interim analysis of a phase three study (Hera study), which demonstrated a therapeutic benefit of around 50 per cent for patients with early HER2 positive breast cancer (Breast Cancer International Research Group, 2005). The Hera Study demonstrated that following one year of Trastuzumab 92.5 per cent of patients were disease free compare to 87.1 per cent of the control arm (Paccart-Gebhart et al., 2005). This equated to a 24 per cent reduction in mortality and necessitated the participants in the control arm be offered the opportunity to switch to receiving Trastuzumab. Following this guidance being published our cancer network predicted the Trust would be required to administer Trastuzumab in the adjuvant setting to 25 patients per annum (Northern Cancer Network [NCN], 2006).

Trastuzumab had been used since 2001 as a form of treatment for HER2+ metastatic breast cancer (Pace and Mcllroy, 2004), therefore clinicians were familiar with the possible side effects, including cardiotoxicity, fever and chills, infusion reactions and rarely anaphylaxis (Roche, 2006). The potential side effects to monoclonal antibodies are totally different to those resulting from the administration of chemotherapy, such as alopecia, nausea and vomiting and myelosuppression (Bell, 2002). The NCRI Breast Clinical Studies Group (2005), after reviewing all available evidence, decided that Trastuzumab should be administered in the adjuvant setting within six months of completing adjuvant chemotherapy and at least three weeks after receiving an anthracycline agent. This guidance was in keeping with the results of the Hera study performed by Paccart-Gebhart et al (2005).

The cancer network where I work had already made the decision to offer Trastuzumab to patients with early stage HER2 positive breast cancer, based on the available clinical and cost effective evidence (Northern Cancer Network [NCN], 2005).

When NICE (2006a) issued its guidance on the use of Trastuzumab for HER2+ early breast cancer, it emphasised the importance of cardiac monitoring, which would involve either three monthly echocardiogram (echo) or radionuclide (MUGA) imaging. Our organisation chose to undertake echocardiograms, as they are non-invasive and readily accessible. Cardiac monitoring is necessary since Trastuzumab has the potential to decrease the left ventricular ejection fraction (LVEF) and possibly cause heart failure (Roche, 2006).

The administration of Trastuzumab

Trastuzumab is administered as an infusion every three weeks for one year (NICE, 2006a) and initially was administered over 90 minutes. With increased clinical experience and monitoring of patients the timing was reduced to 30 minutes in 2009. As Trastuzumab is a monoclonal antibody there is an increased risk of allergic reaction with the first infusion, therefore national recommendations were to monitor patients for six hours from commencement of the first infusion and for a period of two hours following commencement of the second infusion onwards

(NCRI Breast Clinical Studies Group, 2005); this again was something that was also reduced over time.

Initially there was only limited data regarding the use of Trastuzumab in the adjuvant setting, therefore NICE (2006b) recommended auditing clinical use in this setting. This would ensure that their guidance (NICE 2006a) was implemented throughout the England and Wales and compliance was met. NICE (2006b) recommended that hospital trusts should undertake audits for a period of six months periodically, and results were fed into a national database. By completing this audit the organisation would be able to ensure that the clinical benefits by reducing the risk of recurrence was balanced against the treatment costs in this patient group and, importantly, provide an opportunity to monitor side effects that patients experienced (NICE, 2006a).

Rationale for developing a nurse-led pathway

My role requires me to spend a great deal of my clinical sessions managing and caring for patients with breast cancer, as well as being seen as a senior nurse in my organisation, having influence in the cancer setting to drive change (Reid, 2002). As the nominated local lead (National Health Service [NHS], 2005), I was addressing one of the challenges outlined by the Cancer Service Collaborative (CSC, 2005b) in relation to moving tasks/roles up/down traditional unidisciplinary ladders. This enabled me to ensure a greater emphasis was placed on team working and peer support, rather than hierarchical and controlling, which have previously been seen in the Health Service (Department of Health [DOH], 2002b), especially since many may have presumed an oncologist would have led the development. It also offered me the opportunity to expand the breadth and depth of my existing role. By developing this pathway I demonstrated that patient care was provided by appropriately skilled and knowledgeable professionals in the correct and safe setting for the patients, rather than traditional consultant (oncologist) led follow-up (NHS, 2005), which would free up their capacity for other tasks (CSC, 2005b).

Around this time there had been many changes in nursing roles which focused on improving patients' experiences, by providing high quality care that constantly needed to be assessed in order to respond to patients' changing needs (DOH, 2002a). Nurses were able to lead developments and demonstrate their abilities by utilising their skills and knowledge to provide a high quality, safe and effective service locally (DOH, 2002b). An example of such developments in nursing was the introduction of consultant nurses (Manley, 2000) and greater provision of nurse-led services across the cancer setting (CSC, 2005b).

As a consultant nurse I aim to lead nursing locally, nationally and internationally (Hopwood, 2006), demonstrating the fundamental elements of my role, which include strong leadership skills and an acknowledged clinical base, alongside key roles in education and research, which all contribute to being a recognised change agent (Higgins, 2003). Within my role I have shared values and a common purpose with other professionals (Manley, 2000) with functions across many organisational and professional boundaries to ensure continuity, integration and sustainability of services provided for cancer patients (Higgins, 2003).

The Chief Nursing Officer in 2002 outlined 10 key development roles to assist nurses to ultimately improve patient care and be seen as key player in the provision of care delivery through innovation and development of their roles. It also provided an opportunity to rid the Health Service of traditional boundaries that have previously prevented nursing developments. This transition became more evident with the increased blurring of the doctor/nurse boundaries (Redwood et al., 2007) and the introduction of many nurse-led clinics and care pathways (CSC, 2005b).

The development of this multiprofessional patient pathway allowed me to demonstrate seven of the ten Chief Nursing Officer's key roles (DOH, 2002a) in that I order investigations, make and receive referrals, admit and discharge patients when appropriate and in accordance with the agreed pathway, manage my own patient caseload and continue to run nurse-led clinics, which include prescribing Trastuzumab and supportive treatments. Finally, and importantly for my organisation and the Primary Care Trust, my role was recognised by taking the lead in the way cancer care is organised and delivered locally (Redwood et al., 2007), which included decisions regarding resource allocation (DOH, 2002b).

General pathway development

Within the cancer setting there has always been a focus on delivering efficient and patient centred care (Bryan et al., 2002) by utilising clinical guidelines/pathways (Hewitt-Taylor, 2003), which also ensure care is based on available evidence (Hewitt-Taylor, 2006). Clinical guidelines also viewed by many professionals as a way of demonstrating the principles of clinical governance (Reid, 2002), which contribute to providing quality care for patients (Nursing & Midwifery Council, 2004) based on best available evidence rather than traditional or individual professionals' beliefs (Hewitt-Taylor, 2006). They are also seen as a way of eradicating ineffective, inappropriate and potentially dangerous practices (Reid, 2002). A guideline also offers the opportunity to measure practice and provide educations and learning for other professionals (Hewitt-Taylor, 2006). NICE is a national example of an organisation that has responsibility for producing national guidance in relation to ensuring excellence in practice, through the promotion of good health, prevention and treatment of ill health.

Whilst I acknowledged the importance of clinical guidelines/pathways for the above reasons and as a way of ensuring equitable provision of care and helping to minimise 'postcode' care, I was also pleased that NICE acknowledged that guidelines should always be used in conjunction with practitioners' clinical judgement and individual patients' wishes (NICE, 2003). Hewitt-Taylor (2003) cited the example of where a novice nurse would adhere strictly to the guidelines as though 'set in stone', whereas the expert nurse would utilise her clinical experience and knowledge to judge whether the guideline/pathway could be detrimental for individual patients.

The national guidance for Trastuzumab (NICE, 2006a) and the cancer network guidance (NCN, 2006) needed translating into a workable local pathway, which I developed and implemented with the assistance of other key professionals. Optimising my role in terms of utilising my skills and knowledge regarding the treatment of breast cancer enabled me to implement changes in care delivery and team working, to develop a pathway that would improve care, reduce waste and/or duplication, improve working lives and benefit patient care (NHS, 2005).

Development and implementation of the Trastuzumab pathway

Previously there had been no defined pathway for patients receiving Trastuzumab, whether in the metastatic or adjuvant setting. This meant patients were seen in routine cardiology clinics where the staff were not aware of the importance of the ejection faction in terms of whether the patient received treatment or not. In 2009 I initiated the development of the pathway due to concerns about the management of patients receiving Trastuzumab.

I had previously utilised the step-by-step guide to developing protocols produced by the NHS Modernisation Agency and NICE (2004) as a basis for changing practice. All the steps are not necessarily required for all developments; however I found the process assisted in the development of this pathway. Step one of the guide outlines the need to establish the topic which a protocol would address, which in this instance incorporated the NICE guidance in relation to Trastuzumab for patients with HER2+ early breast cancer (NICE, 2006a). This provided the supportive evidence to assist in the implementation of this new treatment option.

Step two of the guide (NHS Modernisation Agency and NICE, 2004) outlined the importance of involving other key professionals early in the process. This process remains important within cancer care due to an increase in the number of professionals involved in a patient's care and the complexity of the treatment options available (Fleissig et al., 2006). However, I was also aware of numerous other service frameworks and initiatives for other professional groups involved with this pathway (Hewitt-Taylor, 2006) that are not cancer-related but equally as important.

Teamwork is considered to be a key component of any effective organisational change (NHS Modernisation Agency, 2003). I learnt through previous experience, both in leading and involvement in multiprofessional initiatives, that the only way for changes to succeed and be sustainable is to involve all professional groups affected by the change (Kenny, 2002). This will minimise the risk of failure due to poor communication, lack of coordination and interprofessional resistance, all of which would have a negative impact on the delivery of patient care (Freir et al., 2004).

I was able to share the evidence supporting the necessity for the pathway (NICE, 2006a) with other key professionals (Reid, 2002), which created an opportunity to debate issues regarding pathway development and implementation (NHS Modernisation Agency, 2003). I also ensured ongoing effective multiprofessional working (Kenny, 2002), which would also demonstrate recognition of the varying knowledge and skills of the team members (Hewitt-Taylor, 2006) and their roles in the pathway (NHS Modernisation Agency, 2003).

I was in a fortunate position, having worked jointly with the pharmacy and the cardiology teams in both hospitals on previous care pathways, to have already developed two-way trust and a respectful working relationship with both teams (NHS Modernisation Agency, 2003). At the time I had not worked directly with the pathology department on implementing changes to practice, although we participated in multidisciplinary team meetings together. The key requirements of the NICE guidance (NICE, 2006a) were used to produce a local pathway in 2009 with the assistance of all involved professionals (see Table 9.1).

The implementation of the pathway met the fourth step of the step-by-step guide to developing protocols (NHS Modernisation Agency and NICE, 2004) by agreeing to key objectives. This would also be viewed as a learning opportunity for all involved, especially since multidisciplinary consultations and management

Table 9.1 Developing the Trastuzumab pathway

Requirement:	Professional group:
Request for tumour to be HER2 tested following surgery	Breast team
Confirmed histology showing early HER2 positive breast cancer	Histopathology (local and network centre)
Patient appropriate to receive Trastuzumab	Oncologist
Pre cardiac assessment using echo demonstrating: • Left ventricular ejection fraction greater than 55% • No evidence of congestive cardiac failure • Not at high risk of uncontrolled arrhythmias • No angina pectoris requiring medication • No clinically significant valvular disease • No evidence of infarction • No poorly controlled hypertension	Cardiology (consultant and technicians)
Baseline bloods: • Full blood count (Fbc) • Urea & Electrolytes (U&Es) • Liver function tests (LFTs) – to demonstrate no liver metastases	Nurses – take bloods Porter – deliver samples Pathology – analyse samples
Check all results and organise 1st prescription of Trastuzumab	Consultant nurse oncologist

(Continued)

Table 9.1 (Continued)

Requirement:	Professional group:
Prescribe Trastuzumab and other medication	Consultant nurse
Reconstitution of Trastuzumab	Aseptic pharmacists
Delivery of Trastuzumab	Porter
Administration of pre medication and loading dose of Trastuzumab. Patient to be monitored for 6 hours from commencing infusion (cycle 1)	Nurse – administer drug Chair – 6 hours
Prescribe Trastuzumab and other medication	Consultant nurse
Reconstitution of Trastuzumab	Aseptic pharmacists
Delivery of Trastuzumab	Porter
Administration of pre medication and maintenance dose of Trastuzumab. Patient to be monitored for 2 hours from commencing infusion (Cycle 2)	Nurse – administer drug Chair – 2 hours
Prescribe Trastuzumab and other medication	Consultant nurse
Reconstitution of Trastuzumab	Aseptic pharmacists
Delivery of Trastuzumab	Porter
Administration of pre medication and maintenance dose of Trastuzumab. (Cycle 3–18)	Nurse – administer drug Chair – 1½ hours
Cardiac assessment (echo) every three months whilst receiving Trastuzumab	Cardiology (consultant and technicians)
Bloods – every three months whilst receiving Trastuzumab •FBC •U&Es •LFTs – to demonstrate no liver metastases	Nurses – take bloods Porter – deliver samples Pathology – analyse samples
Clinical assessment (after cycle 1, 2, 3, then every three months following echo, or sooner if required)	Consultant cancer nurse
Refer patient back to breast team for routine follow up and provide treatment information for patients General Practitioner	Consultant nurse Breast team General practitioner
Post-Trastuzumab cardiac assessment at 3, 6, 12 & 24 months	Cardiology (consultant and technicians)
Collection of audit data for each treatment of each patient (for organisation and Primary Care Trust for funding)	Consultant nurse Senior pharmacist

were considered essential to the current health care system (Fleissig et al., 2006). By implementing this pathway the team would be able to demonstrate how professional groups can work collectively and equally (Kenny, 2002) for the benefit of the patient and the organisation (Frier et al., 2004). This pathway offered the different professional groups an opportunity to demonstrate teamwork across professional disciplines where they shared responsibilities. The professionals were dependant on each other to make the pathway work effectively and were all accountable for its implementation and ultimate success (NHS Modernisation Agency, 2003).

As part of the pathway implementation process I organised a number of study evenings, which all professional groups were invited to participate. The sessions included an update on the management of breast cancer provided by the oncologist, an overview of the mechanisms of Trastuzumab (Roche, 2006) and the supportive evidence behind the NICE guidance (NICE, 2006a), along with a session provided by myself relating to the development and implementation of the pathway. The sessions were very well attended and I felt privileged to actually know and have worked with all the participants.

The need to assess capacity and demand

The NHS Modernisation Agency and NICE (2004) highlighted the importance of conducting a baseline assessment of what impact the planned changes may have on the existing service and any current shortfalls which would need addressing. This was an important consideration in relation to implementing Trastuzumab since it was a new treatment option rather than a replacement for an existing treatment. Therefore I needed to establish the potential demand for the treatment as well as establishing whether existing capacity would meet this demand. This exercise provided the basis for undertaking a capacity and demand exercise; a process that I had needed to repeat on numerous occasions when introducing any changes in practice.

Chemotherapy services are continually changing due to newer treatment options becoming available (Shield, 2004), which in turn place a greater demand for clinical services and an increase in workloads (Summerhayes, 2003). Some of the factors which have influenced this include patients living longer more chemotherapy being administered in the adjuvant and metastatic settings and an increase in the number of lines of treatment in certain tumour types (Summerhayes, 2003). In addition, many of the traditional inpatient regimens are now administered in the outpatient setting since this is more convenient for patients; also the complexities of regimens have increased along with some infusion times (Delaney et al., 2002)

The increase in demand for chemotherapy and use of monoclonal antibodies (Dikken and Smith, 2006), including Trastuzumab, has led to increased workload and stress amongst health professionals due to the overwhelming impact of such treatments (Delaney et al., 2002), and waiting lists have developed in some areas, due to limited resources and physical capacity to provide the required service within current chemotherapy units (Summerhayes, 2003). However, the increase in demand has not necessarily been reflected in an increase in staffing levels and facilities (Dikken and Smith, 2006; Sheild, 2004), and this still remains a familiar occurrence in 2015.

Prior to the planned change of introducing Trastuzumab for early HER2+ breast cancer patients within the current service, we had to undertake an internal capacity and demand study. Dicken and Smith (2006) state the importance of this process in offering the opportunity of reviewing the current service and produce required evidence, which in this case would assist in the submission of a business case to secure additional funding. Also, capacity and demand studies are a national requirement in cancer settings (Department of Health, 2004).

The Institute for Innovations and Improvement in 2005 described the process of matching available capacity, including all available resources. This included staff, space, chairs and 'chair time' to match the predicted demand or number of referrals for the service, and was achieved by defining the group of patients with HER2+ breast cancer who would be affected by the change. Emphasis was also placed on the importance of identifying and involving all key professionals, which would include histology/pathology, cardiology, nursing, pharmacy and medical colleagues.

In the same year the CSC (2005a) produced a capacity-planning tool to assist health professionals capture data on capacity and demand. This tool was developed to address the many challenges being faced nationally by chemotherapy services, and followed the key principles from the Institute for Innovations and Improvement (2005). The process involved using a national chemotherapy administration capacity-planning tool, which produced timing for all chemotherapy regimens from the patient arriving, receiving their treatment through to leaving the department, therefore providing the overall demand for the service. Due to national benchmarking of these times, different services and cancer networks could compare their own workloads and ways of working (DOH, 2004).

The tool also examines capacity offered by the service in terms of the level of nurse available and their availability (in hours) to administer chemotherapy along with the amount of time (in hours) that chemotherapy administration chairs are needed per chemotherapy regimen (see Figures 9.1 and 9.2).

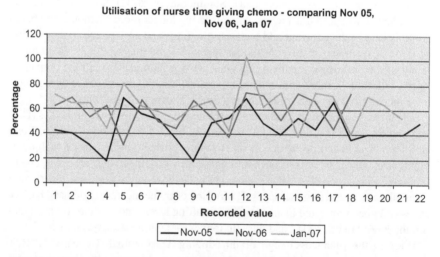

Figure 9.1 Utilisation of nursing time administering chemotherapy

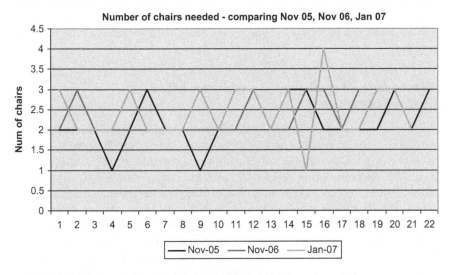

Figure 9.2 Requirements for chemotherapy chairs

Table 9.2 Capacity impact across all clinical areas

Resource item	Current utilisation (days)	Utilisation with planned practice (days)	Marginal impact (days)
Nurse time	0	40	Extra 40 days required
Pharmacy time	0	20	Extra 20 days required
Chair time	0	90	Extra 90 days required

The results of my capacity study indicated that, based on the head of population (330,000 people in 2009) served by our Trust, approximately 50 breast cancer patients would require Trastuzumab in the adjuvant setting. This was double predicted figures from the local cancer network (Northern Cancer Network, 2006), and has shown to be a more accurate prediction. This highlighted the need for local data collection to accurately predict clinical requirements. This figure of 50 patients receiving Trastuzumab over 12 months would require an additional 40 nursing hours and 90 chair hours (see Table 9.2). In addition I had to take into account other developments within the service which were occurring at the same time.

All the data relating to the demand for Trastuzumab and the capacity to deliver the service at a local level helped me to produce a business case for additional funding to include staffing and additional resources. This also included pharmacy and cardiology data to support the provision of their services within the new pathway.

Trastuzumab pathway six months after implementation

Six months following the successful development and implementation of the pathway there were 36 patients registered at various points, which raised questions about the original predictions. All of the patients received regular cardiac assessment, including monitoring their blood profile and clinical assessment, which I conducted (NICE, 2006a). At this point I had managed all the patients in terms of side effects with the exception of one patient who was withdrawn from the pathway due to cardiotoxicity which required long-term management by the heart failure team.

The pathway demonstrated how various professional groups could work together in achieving one common goal to benefit patient care, improve working relationships and communication (Freir et al., 2004). From a personal perspective the pathway offered me the opportunity to develop my role as an independent prescriber and receive recognition (Hopson, 2006) by colleagues, my organisation and the Primary Care Trust for leading the pathway developments (Higgins, 2003) and also for developing nursing within cancer care and demonstrating that nurses can lead clinical initiatives as well as doctors (NHS, 2005).

The pathway was jointly evaluated by the all the key professionals, which is one of the final steps in the step-by-step guide (NHS Modernisation Agency and NICE, 2004). Only minor changes were required, such as only requesting an echo pre-treatment, and then the cardiology team would book subsequent echocardiograms. Also the pathology service was streamlined to speed up the time taken to receive HER2 results from the regional centre in Newcastle.

Due to my perseverance in producing the audit data, preparing other treatment pathways and business cases, along with attending many meetings, both within my organisation and the local Primary Care Trust I was also successful in securing funding for an additional chemotherapy nurse, which was the only additional member to our nursing team

I have continued to use the step-by-step guide to developing protocols/guidelines (NHS Modernisation Agency and NICE, 2004), despite other tools becoming available as I feel it is easy to understand and explain to other professional. More importantly it follows a logical format and is helpful in achieving the required outcomes in a busy clinical environment at a local level.

2010: Introduction of the first combined cardiology/oncology clinic in the UK

In 2010 my cardiology colleagues and I introduced the first combined clinic, which was a huge step forward locally and nationally. It offered the opportunity to ensure adherence to current NICE guidance for cardiac monitoring by echocardiogram or radionuclide (MUGA) imaging (NICE, 2006b). Our organisation utilises echocardiograms as a standard form of monitoring and only uses MUGA's where images are unacceptable on echocardiogram, for example a breast implant.

A key part of this clinic was that it provided an opportunity to meet patients following their final cycle of chemotherapy. This enabled me to explain greater detail about Trastuzumab, such as its difference to chemotherapy, method and duration of administration, possible side effects, the need for continued cardiac monitoring and potential eligibility for clinical trials. During radiotherapy treatment patients also meet a member of the clinical trials team who supports recruitment for the Persephone study, which compares 6 months versus 12 months of Trastuzumab for early breast cancer (Warwick Medical School, 2011).

When attending the clinic patients meet both myself and the cardiologist who performed the echocardiogram / provided a cardiac assessment. These appointments also provided an opportunity for further discussion regarding Trastuzumab and to answer any questions patients may have. Patients often asked questions about side effects from endocrine treatment in addition to Trastuzumab. On leaving the clinic patients would have an appointment for Trastuzumab administration, which at the time was given intravenously, their next cardiology appointment, and with my contact details. A member of the clinical trials team was available for if the patient expressed an interest in the Persephone study (Warwick Medical School, 2011) from the beginning of their treatment and if so I would complete the recruitment process. If patients decided to enter the study at a later date a member of the trials team and I would meet them during one of their treatment appointments. The pathway continues throughout the patient's treatment with Trastuzumab and for two year following treatment, which offers patient continuity, although appointments became less frequent.

One difficulty when implementing this pathway was that my organisation includes two hospitals 40 miles apart, and as the clinic was delivered in one hospital, this meant difficult journeys for many patients. Over time it became apparent that the number of patients accessing the pathway were split 50:50 between the two hospitals, which meant half of the patients drove an 80-mile round trip for their echocardiogram, yet this could be performed locally. Patients questioned why they couldn't have this appointment in the other hospital, which already provides chemotherapy review clinics, and the cardio-physiologist also works across both sites. This one change would save patients unnecessary travel and also release capacity at the main hospital which was struggling to meet cardiology demands

The cardiologist involved in setting up the combined clinic left the organisation in 2011, which meant the format of the clinic needed to change. Following a number of discussions between the team the echocardiograms are now performed by a cardio-physiologist, whilst patient review continued to be undertaken by myself and a cardiologist is available for advice if required. The changes did not compromise patient care and there was a decrease in the clinic costs (Roe, 2014).

Service demands continued to increase, partly due to gastric patients also requiring cardiac monitoring whilst receiving Trastuzumab (Roche, 2013). Therefore, before implementing any further changes I wanted to determine patients' opinions of the current service and the possible changes, which may be considered.

2012: Trastuzumab pathway evaluation from patients' perspective

I developed a patient satisfaction survey to determine whether the pathway met patients' needs and opinions regarding possible future developments (Roe, 2014). Thirty-two out of 40 patients who were either accessing or had recently accessed the pathway completed the survey, which was a good response rate. The survey included a number of closed questions along with a free text box with each question for additional comments and a section for general feedback. Some of the questions focused on receiving the Trastuzumab, which at the time was given as an infusion, the timing of the infusion and satisfaction with the overall pathway. The results demonstrated a positive account of the pathway and this influenced future changes with the pathway and combined clinic.

The questions focused on the following aspects of the pathway:

> *Provision of information received prior to commencing Trastuzumab*: The majority of patients felt they did (see Figure 9.3), however some felt they would have liked further information regarding side effects and management strategies.
> *Where would you prefer your echocardiogram performing?* This question resulted in roughly an equal split between the two hospitals, which were representative of the patient split (see Figure 9.4). I felt that by altering the format of the original clinic, i.e. reducing the number of appointments and initiating an equal number of appointments at the other hospital, the clinic would meet the needs of patients and better utilise available capacity in both hospitals.

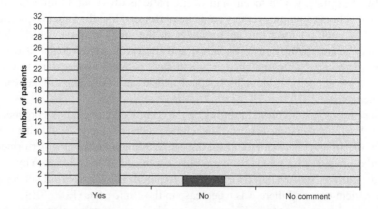

Figure 9.3 Provision of information prior to commencing Trastuzumab

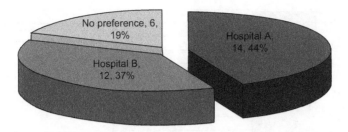

Figure 9.4 Where would you prefer your echocardiogram to be performed?

Where you offered the opportunity to take part in a clinical trial? The clinical trials team actively screens all patients and we discuss the Persephone study (Warwick Medical School, 2011) with all eligible patients, therefore the response to this question was reassuring, as was the number of patients recruited.

Choice of place to receive Trastuzumab: Given the capacity issues for both nursing and pharmacy services, one possible option was for the patients to receive their treatment (after initial two cycles) in the community delivered by an independent trained chemotherapy nursing service. However, the majority of patients preferred to receive their treatment in a hospital setting (see Figure 9.5). Nevertheless I felt that patients should be given a choice regarding this.

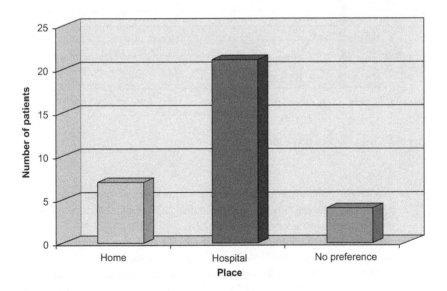

Figure 9.5 Choice of place to receive Trastuzumab

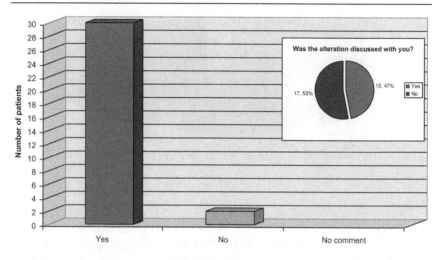

Figure 9.6 Length of infusion reduced to 30 minutes

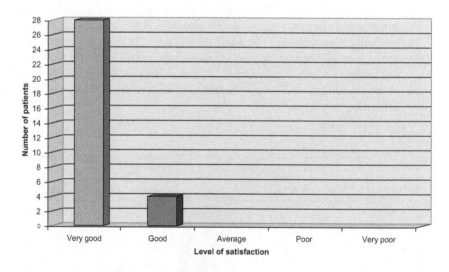

Figure 9.7 Overall satisfaction with service

Length of the infusion time: At the time there was a national consensus to reduce the infusion time from 90 minutes to 30 minutes from cycle two if the patient has no allergic reactions.

The results showed compliance with this in the majority of cases, releasing nursing and chair time. However the survey showed that half the patients had no recollection of discussions regarding this option (see Figure 9.6).

Overall satisfaction with the pathway: The results to this question were very pleasing as they mirrored verbal reports from patients (see Figure 9.7).

The positive response rate to the survey provided a great deal of information that helped to ensure that the pathway remained patient focused. Patients also highlighted areas for improvement such as travel and the inconvenience when drugs arrived late from pharmacy.

Following this patient feedback the clinic was restructured to provide a service on both hospital sites and the team continues to offer and recruit patients into clinical trials in particular the Persephone study (Warwick Medical School, 2011). Discussion also took place with the pharmacy department around time patients waited for their treatment.

2014: Switching from intravenous to subcutaneous administration

The next key development in the pathway came when NHS England approved the use of Trastuzumab as a subcutaneous formulation, with hyaluronidase as an excipient for HER2+ breast cancer (NHS England, 2013), followed by a successful application to extend the product license for Trastuzumab to include a subcutaneous formulation (NICE, 2013).

This application was based on the evidence of the HannaH study, which compared the pharmacokinetic profile, efficacy and safety of subcutaneous and intravenous formulations. The results demonstrated non-inferiority with subcutaneous Trastuzumab, therefore subcutaneous administration should be considered as a valid option, especially considering the potential benefits for patient in terms of convenience (Ismael et al., 2012) since the administration of subcutaneous Trastuzumab only takes five minutes, and is a less invasive procedure. There are also a number of clinical resource implications for clinical practice since the subcutaneous formulation is a standard dose, in contrast to the intravenous preparation, which is calculated on individual patient's weight; also subcutaneous Trastuzumab does not need reconstituting, which requires less pharmacy, nursing and chair time (Ismeal et al., 2012). This demonstrates clear opportunities for cost savings and reductions in capacity (Burcombe et al., 2013).

The PrefHer study also demonstrated that patients preferred to receive Trastuzumab subcutaneously (single-use injection devise or handheld syringe) rather than intravenously. (Pivot et al., 2013). The ongoing SafeHer study continues to assess the safety and tolerability of assisted and self-administration of the subcutaneous Trastuzumab injection (Clinicaltrials.gov, 2014). The results of this study will be vital when developing future services and deciding the most appropriate setting for the injections to be administered and by whom.

Cardiac monitoring for subcutaneous Trastuzumab remains the same as intravenous, requiring patients to have an echo or MUGA every three months whilst receiving treatment and every six months following treatment for two years (Roche, 2014), although some centres undertake cardiac assessments less frequently, particularly post completion of Trastuzumab where the LVEF has been within normal limits.

A United Kingdom time and motion study (Burcombe et al., 2013) was undertaken alongside the PrefHer study to quantify the time and costs associated with intravenous and subcutaneous methods of administering Trastuzumab. This identified substantial savings in terms of time, consumables and overall costs from switching to subcutaneous administration.

Implications of switching to subcutaneous administration in practice

In our organisation all existing patients were offered the opportunity to switch, including those participating in the Persephone study (Warwick Medical School, 2011), although some chose not to switch if they only had a few treatments remaining. All new patients were commenced on the subcutaneous formulation. Interestingly no patients asked to switch back to intravenous Herceptin and all appear very happy with service provided.

When the license was granted for the subcutaneous formulation to be used in practice it recommended that patients were monitored for six hours after the first injection and two hours after subsequent injections. However this created capacity issues in our treatment areas, therefore I approached our Trust drugs and therapeutics committee to request a reduction in the post-injection observation period since there was no post-observation period during clinical trials. The committee agreed an observation period of two hours after the first injection with no observation period after subsequent injections, providing I audited patients' side effects.

2014: Auditing the switch for reported side effects

To address this I undertook an audit for three months from 1 March 2014 to 30 June 2014. This included 17 patients aged 38–71 years, with both adjuvant and metastatic treatments, who received 75 subcutaneous Trastuzumab injections in total (see Figure 9.8). This group included patients switching from an intravenous to subcutaneous formulation, those commencing first-cycle Trastuzumab in a subcutaneous form, and patients receiving Trastuzumab as a single agent or in combination with another systemic anti-cancer treatment such as chemotherapy.

The audit results demonstrated the following:

- One instance of heart failure
- Two instances of skin reactions at and around the injection site which appeared a few days after the injection and lasted for 24–48 hours
- Two instances of flu-like symptoms; Paracetamol was administered with future injections as would have been the case with intravenous Trastuzumab
- Two instances of diarrhoea (manageable) around 5–7 days post-injection

Other than the skin reactions the side effects reported were similar to those seen with intravenous Trastuzumab. The audit results indicated that switching to subcutaneous Trastuzumab had brought many benefits for patients in terms of less

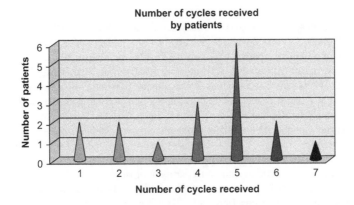

Figure 9.8 Evaluation of switching to subcutaneous Trastuzumab

time spent in the hospital, no need for cannulation and similar side effects to the intravenous preparation. In terms of service delivery the switch has freed up much needed capacity, reduced nursing and pharmacy time, minimised drug wastage and increased flexibility with scheduling treatments. I have continually involved patients in decision-making from pre-switch, through treatment and evaluation. The audit also suggested that the proposed reduction in observation was satisfactory since the reported side effects would not have been prevented by a longer observation period.

Current situation regarding the pathway

The pathway is now well embedded in practice across the various disciplines within our organisation, and patients continue to be involved in decisions about their care. This was evident when deciding a switch strategy based on patients' preferences rather than the decision to switch on a certain date. Patient involvement has been vital in all aspects of development and ongoing monitoring of the pathway to evaluate their experience.

I am currently undertaking a time and motion study to demonstrate the potential savings from switching to the subcutaneous formulation and the impact on clinical practice. Discussions are now being held to determine whether treatments should be given in the community to reduce patient travel and increase capacity in clinical areas. However, continuity will be maintained since patients will still attend the combined cardiology clinic where I am present.

References

Bell R. (2002). 'What can we learn from Herceptin trials in metastatic breast cancer?' *Oncology*. 63: S39–46.

Breast Cancer International Research Group (2005). *Interim analysis of phase III study show docetaxel-based chemotherapy regimes combined with Trastuzumab significantly improved disease free survival in early stage HER2 positive breast cancer.* Proceedings from the 28th annual San Antonio Breast Cancer Symposium. Abstract #1.

Bryan S., Holmes S., Postlethwaite D. & Carty N. (2002). 'The role of integrated care pathways in improving the patient experience'. *Professional Nurse.* 18(2): 77–79.

Burcombe R., Chan S., Simcock R., Samantra K., Percival F. & Barrett-Lee P. (2013). Abstract P4–12–23: Subcutaneous Trastuzumab (Herceptin) in patients with HER-2 positive early breast cancer: a UK time and motion study in comparison with intravenous formulation. *Cancer Research.* 73: 12–23.

Cancer Service Collaborative (2005a). *Chemotherapy service improvement – modernising chemotherapy services – a practical guide to redesign.* London, Department of Health.

Cancer Service Collaborative (2005b). *Applying high impact changes to cancer care – excellence in cancer care.* London, Department of Health.

ClinicalTrials.gov (2014). A safety and tolerability study of assisted and self assisted administrated subcutaneous Herceptin (Trastuzumab) as adjuvant therapy in patients with early HER2-postive breast cancer (SafeHer). Available at: www.clinicaltrials.gov/show/NCT01566721

Department of Health (2004). *Manual of cancer service standards.* London, Department of Health.

Department of Health (2002a). *Developing key roles for nurse and midwives – a guide for managers.* London, Department of Health.

Department of Health (2002b). *Shifting the balance of power: the next steps.* London, Department of Health.

Delaney G., Bin J., Moylan E. & Barton M. (2002). 'The development of a model of outpatient chemotherapy delivery – chemotherapy basic treatment equivalent (CBTE)'. *Cancer Oncology.* 14: 406–412.

Dikkens C. & Smith K. (2006). 'Calculating capacity and demand in chemotherapy outpatient units.' *Cancer Nursing Practice.* 5(8): 35–39.

Fleissig A., Jenkins V., Catt S. & Fallowfield L. (2006). 'Multidisciplinary teams in cancer care: are they effective in the UK?' *Lancet Oncology.* 7: 935–943.

Freir V., Gordon M., Richmond J. & Wheeler D. (2004). 'The jigsaw puzzle of a multidisciplinary team. *Cancer Nursing Practice.* 3(3): 19–21.

Hopwood L. (2006). 'Developing advanced nursing practice roles in cancer care'. *Nursing Times.* 102(15): S4–5.

Higgins A. (2003). 'The developing role of the consultant nurse'. *Nursing Management.* 10(1): 22–28.

Hewitt-Taylor J. (2006). *Clinical care guidelines and care protocols.* Chichester, John Wiley & Sons.

Hewitt-Taylor J. (2003). 'Developing and using clinical guidelines'. *Nursing Standard.* 18(5): 41–44.

Institute for Innovation and Improvement (2005). *Improvement leaders' guide – matching capacity and demand.* Nottingham, National Health Service Institute for Innovation and Improvement.

Ismael G., Hegg R., Susanne S., Heinzmann D., Lum B., Kim S.B., Pienkowski T., Lichinitser M., Semiglazov V., Melichar B., Jackisch C. (2012). Subcutaneous versus intravenous administration of (neo)adjuvant trastuzumab in patients with HER2-positive, clinical stage I–III breast cancer (HannaH study): a phase 3, open-label, multicentre, randomised trial. *The Lancet Oncology.* 13: 869–878.

Kenny G. (2002). 'Interprofessional working: opportunities and challenges'. *Nursing Standard*. 17(6): 33–35.

Manley K. (2000). 'Organisational culture and consultant nurse outcomes: part 1 organisational culture'. *Nursing Standard*. 24(1): 34–38.

NHS England (2013). *NHS England sanctions new breast cancer treatment injection.* Available at: www.england.nhs.uk/2013/09/24/cancer-treatment-injctn/

National Health Service (NHS) Modernisation Agency & National Institute for Clinical Excellence (NICE) (2004). *A step by step guide to developing protocols.* London, Department of Health.

National Health Service (NHS) Modernisation Agency (2003). *The clinicians' guide to applying the 10 high impact changes.* London, Department of Health.

National Health Service (NHS) Modernisation Agency (2005). *Teamwork for improvement: planning for spread and sustainability.* London, Department of Health.

National Institute for Clinical Excellence (NICE) (2003). *Factsheet: general information about clinical guidelines.* National Institute for Clinical Excellence. London, NICE.

National Institute for Health and Clinical Excellence (NICE) (2006a). *Trastuzumab for the adjuvant treatment of early stage HER2-postive breast cancer.* National Institute for Health and Clinical Excellence. London, NICE.

National Institute for Health and Clinical Excellence (NICE) (2006b). Audit criteria – *Trastuzumab for the adjuvant treatment of early stage HER2-postive breast cancer.* National Institute for Health and Clinical Excellence. London, NICE.

National Institute for Clinical Excellence (NICE) (2013). *ESNM13 Early and metastatic HER2-positive breast cancer: subcutaneous trastuzumab.* Available at: http://www.nice.org.uk/mpc/evidencesummariesnewmedicines/ESNM13.jsp

National Statistics (2005). Available at: http://www.statistics.gov.uk

National Cancer Research Institute Breast Clinical Studies Group *UK clinical guidelines for the use of adjuvant Trastuzumab (Herceptin) with or following chemotherapy in HER2-positive early breast cancer.* Anticancer agents and cardiotoxicity. *Semin Oncol.* 33: 2–14.

NCRI Breast Clinical Studies Group. (2005). UK clinical guidelines for the use of adjuvant trastuzumab (Herceptin) with or following chemotherapy in HER2-positive early breast cancer. http://www.dh.gov.uk/prod_consum_dh/groups/dh_digitalassets/@dh/@en/documents/digitalasset/dh_4126384.pdf [Last accessed 29.07.2015].

Northern Cancer Network (NCN) (2005). *NCN: introduction of adjuvant herceptin for early breast cancer.* Gateshead and Sunderland, Northern Cancer Network.

Northern Cancer Network (NCN) (2006). *Network guidance for the assessment of cardiac function in patients receiving Trastuzumab (Herceptin) drug treatment for HER2-positive breast cancer.* Gateshead and Sunderland, Northern Cancer Network.

Nursing & Midwifery Council (2004). *The NMC Code of Professional Conduct: standards for conduct, performance and ethics.* London, Nursing & Midwifery Council.

Pace E. & McIlory P. (2004). 'Nurse management of Trastuzumab for patient with breast cancer'. *Cancer Nursing Practice.* 3(1): 35–39.

Piccart-Gebhart M., Proctor M., Leyland-Jones B., Goldhirsch A., Untch M., Smith I., Gianni L., Baselga J., Bell R., Jackisch R., Cameron D., Dowsett M., Barrios C., Steger G., Huang C., Andersson M., Inbar M., Lichinitser M., Lang I., Nitz U., Iwata H., Thomssen C., Lohrisch C., Suter T., Ruschoff J., Suto T., Greatorex V., Ward C., Straehle C., McFadden E., Dolci S. & Gelber R. (2005). 'Trastuzumab after adjuvant chemotherapy in HER2 positive breast cancer'. *New England Journal of Medicine*. 353: 1659–1672.

Pivot X., Gligorov J., Müller V., Barrett-Lee P., Verma S., Knoop A., Curigliano G., Semiglazov V., López-Vivanco G., Jenkins V., Scotto N., Osborne S. & Fallowfield L. (2013). 'Preference for subcutaneous or intravenous administration of trastuzumab in patients with HER2 positive early breast cancer (PrefHer): an open-label randomized study'. *Lancer Oncology*. 14(10): 962–970.

Quinn M. (2005). 'Breast'. In *Cancer Atlas of the United Kingdom and Ireland 1991–2000* (M. Quinn, H. Wood, N. Cooper & S. Rowan, eds.) Chapter 5. London. Palgrave Macmillan.

Redwood S., Lloyd H., Carr E., McSherry R., Campbell S. & Graham I. (2007). 'Evaulating nurse consultants' work through key informant perceptions'. *Nursing Standard*. 21(17): 35–40.

Reid W. (2002). 'Clinical governance: implementing a change in workplace practice'. *Professional Nurse*. 17(12): 734–737.

Roche (2006). *Estimating the capacity impact of Roche Oncology Products*. Basel, Roche Products Limited.

Roche (2013). *Herceptin – SPC*. Available at: http://www.medicines.org.uk/emc/medicine/3567/SPC/Herceptin+150mg+Powder+for+concentrate+for+solution+for+infusion/

Roche (2014). *Herceptin – SPC*. Available at: http://www.emc.medicines.org.uk.

Roe H. (2014). Patient's perception of a nurse-led Trastuzumab pathway. *Ecancermedicalscience* 8:419. DOI: 10.3332/ecancer.2014.419

Shield K. (2004). 'Capacity planning for chemotherapy'. *The Pharmaceutical Journal*. 272: 61–62.

Summerhayes M. (2003). 'The impact of workload changes and staff availability on IV chemotherapy services'. *Journal of Oncology Pharmacy Practice*. 9: 123–128.

Warwick Medical School (2011). *Persephone*. Available at: http://www2.warwick.ac.uk/fac/med/research/ctu/trials/cancer/persephone/

Index